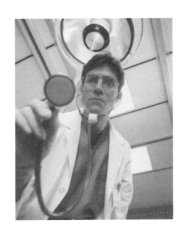

What Your
DOCTOR
Really Thinks

Diagnosing the Doctor-Patient Relationship

Ian Blumer, M.D.

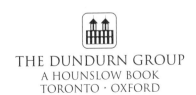

THE DUNDURN GROUP
A HOUNSLOW BOOK
TORONTO · OXFORD

Publisher: Anthony Hawke
Editor: Barry Jowett
Design: Jennifer Scott
Printer: Transcontinental Printing Inc.

Canadian Cataloguing in Publication Data
Blumer, Ian
What your doctor really thinks: diagnosing the doctor-patient relationship
ISBN 0-88882-215-4
1. Physician and patient. 2. Medical ethics. I. Title.
R727.3.B56 1999   610.69'6   C99-932275-3

1   2   3   4   5   03   02   01   00   99

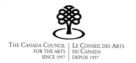

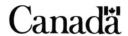

We acknowledge the support of the **Canada Council for the Arts** for our publishing program. We also acknowledge the support of the **Ontario Arts Council** and the financial support of the Government of Canada through the **Book Publishing Industry Development Program** (BPIDP) for our publishing activities.

Printed and bound in Canada.

Printed on recycled paper.

Dundurn Press
8 Market Street
Suite 200
Toronto, Ontario, Canada
M5E 1M6

Dundurn Press
73 Lime Walk
Headington, Oxford,
England
0X3 7AD

Dundurn Press
2250 Military Road
Tonawanda, New York
U.S.A. 14150

Table of Contents

For Heather

Introduction

It was during my very first lecture in medical school that I started to learn the truth.

We had timidly made our way into the auditorium, scanning the room for the security of familiar faces amongst our classmates. There were a few smiles of recognition, a few quick waves as we took our seats. Shortly thereafter, Professor Levart entered the room and moved to the podium. He looked up at us, opened his mouth, and **boom**, his voice erupted. Fifteen years later, the explosion still resonates. "So you fooled them, didn't you?!" he bellowed. We sat mute. "Year after year it happens. You guys (*though gals were indeed present*) somehow manage to get adequate marks, connive your way through an interview, twist somebody's arm for a reference and here you are." He paused — I assumed for dramatic effect. "Future doctors. Jesus."

I looked at my neighbour. He looked at me. Nervous laughter. *He's joking, right?* Maybe wrong. You see, many (probably most) of us felt we were gross over-achievers and, as such, believed we truly had fooled our way into medical school. Not with bribes, but with undeservedly good marks. Sure, we knew we weren't dumb, but maybe long hours of study had covered up for lack of intellectual brilliance. We hadn't actually lied to get in, but playing on our insecurities the prof's words sure made us feel we had.

We *had* fooled them. And he knew. And the other profs probably knew. And that was just the start. For soon thereafter we started being trained to fool our patients also.

Sometimes it was overt, like when our professors would introduce us to patients. "Mrs. Johnson, this is Dr. Blumer." *Dr. Blumer? Who's that? Me? Hell, it's my first week of medical school. My grandmother knows more about medicine than I do.*

Other times it was more subtle, such as when the senior physician would stand at the patient's bedside ostensibly giving us a detailed analysis of the physical examination findings, but unbeknownst to the patient, actually using medical jargon to denounce the patient's obvious mental ineptitude and physical sloth.

Whether with good intentions or bad, we quickly came to realize that we were being trained not only to diagnose and treat (and, on wondrous but rare occasions, to actually heal), but to perform. To act. To play the role of doctor.

And the role playing never stops. Though it may have started in medical school, decades later as you stand at the patient's bedside, it's still with you; still your constant companion .

And every patient's companion also. For if the doctor examining you is performing, surely you have no choice but, for better or worse, to be participant also. The doctor and patient are the players; the examining room the stage. And that is what this book is all about. The roles and games that physicians and patients play. Sometimes knowingly. Sometimes not.

Now I wouldn't want you to miss out on playing the role of physician also. For I learned something else in medical school. Everyone wants to be a doctor. At least some of the time.

One day, my father called to ask what I thought might be causing some chest pain he had developed. I gave him the best answer I could. I told him to see a doctor. He did and he was fine. I thought that would put an end to requests for medical advice, but was I ever wrong. The next night he called again; this time to ask whether his belly pains were due to a bowel problem. I gave his question the degree of thought it deserved (which was none at all) and immediately told him that gee, well, I guess he should see a doctor to find out. The end? Nope.

The calls continued for quite some time, but eventually, I'm happy to say, he came to the realization that I was as stubborn as he was and calls for medical advice ceased. I remember feeling badly for Bell Canada shareholders that fiscal quarter.

A few months passed and when home on Christmas break I went to a family gathering. I guess my reputation had spread for no one asked me for advice. (I hoped that didn't reflect their opinion of my abilities). An uncle of mine did, however, come up to me and say "Ian, don't worry, I'm not going to ask for your advice. I know you won't give any. But," (*uh oh, I thought, here it comes*), "why don't you ask me for my opinion?" *Huh?* "You give me some symptoms and let me figure out the problem."

"Okay," I agreed.

"Well," I said, "let's say you have a sixty-year-old man with difficulty passing his urine and a bit of dribbling after he goes. What might be causing that?"

"An enlarged prostate," he said, looking very proud of himself. His answer was right. (I wondered, had my question hit a bit close to home?)

Well, at that point the cat was out of the bag. Some of my other relatives, having overheard the discussion with my uncle, came running over begging me to quiz them also. Hmmm, quite a reversal of roles; the doctor (or in this case, the medical student) asking the relatives medical questions. Anyhow, that got me to thinking that adults aren't much different from kids: they both like playing doctor.

With that in mind I am going to pepper this book with scenarios which call for you too to play doctor and make up your own mind about how you would handle things.

Nowadays, when I'm playing doctor it is as a specialist in internal medicine. This is, as I will point out in a later chapter, quite a broad specialty encompassing everything from *a*sthma to *z*oster ("shingles"). Chances are, anytime you or someone you know has been admitted to hosptial with a non-surgical problem (such as a stroke, heart attack, or pneumonia), the specialist that you first encountered was an internal medicine consultant (also known as an "internist;" not to be confused — *please!* — with an "intern," which is a newly graduated doctor). Thereafter, depending on the problem, you might be referred to a *sub*-specialist such as a cardiologist, neurologist, and so forth. My particular area of sub-specialty interest is in diabetes and thyroid disease.

I have quite arbitrarily structured this book around certain symptoms that are particularly likely to lead someone to visit the doctor. I do so with reluctance since isolating a symptom from the whole patient is sort of like using separate computer keyboards for consonants and vowels. Nonetheless, it does serve as a reasonable jumping-off point in discussing how doctors approach things.

And I have to add the "official disclaimers":

Official disclaimer number one: All people mentioned in this book have had their names and certain other characteristics changed in order to protect their privacy and anonymity (and to make sure I don't get sued).

Official disclaimer number two: Specific medical advice pertaining to your own care should be obtained from your own physician. Naturally.

Chapter One

FATIGUE, NEUTRALITY, AND GREED

A woman of 38, Mrs. Mary Woods, was referred to me by her family doctor because of persisting fatigue. I ushered her in from the waiting room, introduced myself, and brought her down the short corridor into the examining room.

"Have a seat," I said, gesturing to the chair opposite mine. "So, what brings you to see me today?" I asked.

"Doctor, I'm just plain exhausted. I'm tired *all* the time." Mrs. Woods did indeed look fatigued. "My get up and go just got up and went. From the moment I get up until the moment I get into bed all I want to do is rest. I get maybe a little bit of energy mid-day but I'm a wreck the rest of the time. I wonder if I have Chronic Fatigue Syndrome." She looked at me expectantly.

And I looked back neutrally. At least I sure tried to look neutral. Because I didn't want her to know my secret: I don't like seeing patients whose main complaint is fatigue. Why? Because almost invariably it is due to depression. And when I tell patients that, they usually immediately conclude that I believe they therefore have "nothing wrong" with them (which is transparently not true; depression is very real) and moreover that I have obviously missed the boat and failed to figure out what their true illness is. And then, truth be told, some of these patients conclude I am either incompetent (which my wife tells me really just isn't true) or am "just like the rest of them" — *them* being the vast numbers of doctors who obviously don't really care about the patients they look after, they just want them in and out of the office on a treadmill to help finance their golf club dues (and heck, I don't even play golf; though I do admit to having gone sailing on occasion).

What do you think might be causing Mrs. Wood's tiredness?

1. Chronic Fatigue Syndrome
2. cancer
3. an underactive thyroid gland ("hypothyroidism")
4. don't know yet

Answer: 4. It is impossible to know at this point what is causing her problem. We can make an educated guess, but I can tell you right now that malpractice lawyers love it when doctors make educated guesses. I bet you can figure out why.

So, where do we take things from here? Well, we do what doctors have been doing for hundreds (probably thousands) of years. We get more history — "history" being what the patient tells us (as opposed to "physical," which is the physical examination of the patient).

"Mrs. Wood's, please go on," I said.

"I don't know what else to say," she replied.

This is the tricky part of an interview. To inquire, but not to lead.

"Tell me more about your fatigue," I said. Now all I've basically done is just ask the same thing of her twice. Redundant? Perhaps. But it works. Asking things twice may give the impression of not paying attention to the original answer, but experience proves that patients will almost always elaborate if asked the same thing twice.

"Well, I guess I've felt this way for a year or so. Maybe two years. No ... when I think about it I guess I haven't felt right for longer than that, it must be going on two and a half years or more." Mrs. Woods was worried. Like many people, she believed that a symptom going on for that length of time must be due to some dread disease.

So, was she right? Is there an increased likelihood of a serious disease if fatigue is chronic?

1. yes
2. no
3. maybe

Answer: 2. In fact the longer that someone has had fatigue the less likely it is that there is anything sinister underlying it. As an example, someone is not going to have the luxury of being chronically fatigued if they have metastatic lung cancer.

As Mrs. Woods had paused, I asked her what "fatigue" meant to her. Now you might think this would be self evident. Fatigue is fatigue. Ah, if only the practice of medicine were that straightforward. In reality one person's fatigue is not another's.

"It's exhaustion doctor. Just plain exhaustion."

Whereas tiredness for Mrs. Woods was a sense of exhaustion, for others it might be a lack of interest in things or a feeling of somnolence. The differences can be legion.

Were someone complaining of persisting or recurring somnolence to the point that they were falling asleep at inappropriate times, such as when driving or in the middle of conversation, then it would be imperative to evaluate them for the possibility of:

1. sleep apnea
2. neuroses
3. a chronic viral illness
4. African Sleeping Sickness

Answer: 1. In this condition, affected individuals usually believe they have had a good night's sleep, but in fact are sleeping fitfully, having episodes of terrible snoring (sometimes as loud as a jet plane taking off!) and other periods where they stop breathing altogether. The patient of course would not know this. It is noted indirectly — usually when a patient tells me that their spouse is worried about them. The typical comment is along the lines of "Doc, my wife keeps hitting me in the middle of the night because I stop breathing and she thinks I'm not going to start again." More difficult to sort out is the sleep apnea patient who, as is often the case, cannot tell me if his wife finds that he sometimes stops breathing because she has long ago kicked him out of the bedroom. The snoring was too much for her. One day it would not surprise me if I get simultaneous requests to see both husband and wife for fatigue.

People are often judged by the company they keep. Symptoms are assessed in much the same way. Hence, my next question to Mrs. Woods.

"Mrs. Woods, have you noticed anything else?"

"Yes, I find I can't concentrate on things. And my work is suffering. I'm getting worried that my boss is going to notice. Sometimes it's not too bad and I can put in a couple of good hours but most of the time it's a struggle."

"Anything else?"

"Well, to help you I brought this list with me — it tells you everything."

Do you think such a list is:

1. often helpful
2. always helpful
3. never helpful

Answer: 1. But not for the reasons you might expect. Studies have shown that the greater the number of symptoms a patient has identified on a list the lesser the likelihood of any of them being due to a serious disease. So when I see a long list emerge from a wallet or purse, surprising as it seems, this is often a reassuring finding. The downside of a list is that the symptoms so carefully itemized end up being discussed like a check-list rather than real symptoms experienced by a real person. The important symptoms would invariably have been obtained during the course of the interview anyhow and in such a way that conversation would have allowed more fluid elaboration of the details. Although many a patient fears that they will miss a key finding if it is not written down, in fact that's seldom the case. The overlooked symptom is rarely important.

She tells me of her headaches and her dizziness. Her belly pain and her constipation. Her shortness of breath and her chest pain. Her aching and her stiffness. I interject occasionally but for the most part I simply let her speak. It is a difficult balance. Each and every one of her symptoms could be significant, yet to explore them all in detail would take hours and more importantly could lead to losing the forest for the trees.

As the interview progressed it gradually came out that Mrs. Woods had separated from her husband after an increasingly hostile relationship. She had two children, one of whom was having major problems at school.

With all this information now available, what is the most likely diagnosis?

1. hypothyroidism
2. cancer
3. depression
4. heart disease

Answer: 3.

She was depressed; pure and simple. As my report to the family doctor said; "the chronicity, multiplicity, and nonspecificity of this patient's symptoms are typical of functional complaints." Now what the hell does that mean? Well, basically it means that we have someone with a whole potpourri of chronic, vague complaints which have been present virtually forever yet in whom no "physical" disease has ever developed. Note that a very likely diagnosis was established without my having had to ask her more than a handful of questions and indeed without her even yet having had a physical examination. And not a single blood test or x-ray was done. The moral of the story: the history is the key to diagnosis. *The history.* What the patient tells you. That is where the answers usually lie. Or at the very least, where the clues emerge.

But taking a detailed history is very time consuming. And doctors don't have a lot of time. Or at the very least they don't make a lot of time. Family doctors in fact will often book patients six to ten minutes apart. That is a necessity because of both the number of patients that want to (or, ahem, need to) be seen and because the amount you get paid per patient is not a lot. Most doctors are, to put it bluntly, piece workers. It just happens to be that the pieces are people. So if you want to have a good income (and rest assured, most doctors do, and I make no value judgment here: I too certainly like to make a very nice living) there is a strong impetus to not spend a long time with each patient. Consultants have the luxury of being paid more per patient and so have the opportunity to spend more time with them.

Now if a family doc has allotted six minutes for a patient visit, that is fine when all you have is a sore throat, but if you want to discuss your fatigue, do not be surprised if your doctor's practised look of neutrality is not so convincing. Far better to let the doctor's office know in advance that you have a new problem, what it is and let them try to find a longer appointment for you.

Mr. James Ferguson, like Mrs. Woods, came to see me because he was tired. And like Mrs. Woods he complained of feeling exhausted and worn out. But unlike Mrs. Woods, he'd feel not too badly when he would awaken but by mid-day he had to leave work and rest.

So, does that sparse information give us a significant clue as to the cause of this patient's fatigue?

1. yes
2. no
3. maybe

Answer: 1. The warning lights went on. Mine that is. Okay in the morning, but worse as the day progresses. That is often a clue of some serious pathology lurking. The body is refreshed after a night's sleep but fades quickly thereafter.

"Have you noticed anything else?" I asked him.

"These sweats are driving me crazy," he answered. "Every night around three in the morning I'll wake up drenched. My pyjamas get soaked. It's gotten to the point that I have to roll over to the other side of the bed because its drier there."

What should be the very next question I ask Mr. Ferguson?

1. is he coughing
2. is he having diarrhea
3. does he have a water bed

Answer: 3.

"Do you have a water bed?" I asked. You bet I asked. I had one patient I worked up extensively for the problem of night sweats only to find out he had recently obtained a water bed and liked the thermostat turned up. Way up. I don't like feeling foolish.

"No, no water bed. Same bed as always," he told me.

Sweats. Night sweats. That can be a big problem. Both for the annoyance it represents for the patient and for the sometimes sinister disease that can underlie it. Could Mr. Ferguson have Hodgkin's Disease (a type of lymph gland cancer), I wondered? Or tuberculosis? Or an infection of a heart valve (known as endocarditis)?

I asked him about other symptoms, but few were found. As I continued to talk to Mr. Ferguson, I reminded myself that when I examined him I would have to check carefully for the presence of any swollen lymph glands. I asked Mr. Ferguson to change into an examining gown and I left the room. I went into my private office, pulled a textbook off the shelf and opened it to the section on the different causes of night sweats. And by having done so, I was participating in an age-old secret ritual.

The ritual to which I refer is:

a) a covert way to make up for a deficient knowledge base
b) a nice break from being at the patient's bedside
c) understandably kept secret

Choose 1. a) only
       2. a) and b)
       3. a), b) and c)

Answer: 3. Doctors read about you. We read about you when you are changing into your examining gown. We read about you when you are changing back into your clothes. We read about you when we go into the next room to get a prescription pad. And we read about you when we're in the bathroom. It's true. Some doctors keep a veritable library scattered in the different rooms of their office so that they can readily access some information in a discreet way. Way back when, having recently graduated from medical school and having completed my residency (specialty training), I believed that patients in this age of a well-informed public realized that doctors had need to frequently refer to reference materials. And I was right. People do realize this. Patient **x** knows I have to go back to the books to figure out what is wrong with Patient **y**. And Patient **y** knows I have to go back to the books to figure out what is wrong with Patient **x**. What Patient **x** does not generally want to accept is that I have to go to the books to figure out what is wrong with Patient **x**.

One day I was feeling unwell and went to see my own doctor. "Don, I've noticed my eyes are looking a bit yellow at times. Do you think it could be related to my hemoglobinopathy (a disorder of hemoglobin — the molecule that carries oxygen in the blood)?" I asked him.

"Gee Ian," Don said, I don't know. I'll have to go look it up." And he did. Right in front of me! I couldn't believe it. Didn't he know the answer? Could I trust him with my health if he had to go running to the books? Hey, what kind of doctor was this?

Now, intellectually I recognized that I was actually best off with a doctor who realized his limitations; knew what he knew and equally (or even more) importantly, knew what he did not know. Only a fool of a doctor would pretend to "know it all." Oh, I recognized that well enough. But I was still left with a most uncomfortable feeling. I knew that it was irrational, but it was the way I felt. And recognizing that feeling in myself, I could certainly imagine that my patients might have similar sentiments. Hence, doctors end up trying their best to maintain an air of wisdom that at times outstrips their true knowledge.

When I examined Mr. Ferguson I was dismayed to find that he did indeed have a substantial number of enlarged lymph glands. Actually, "dismayed" probably isn't the best choice of words. I was obviously concerned for Mr. Ferguson's well being yet at the same time I was pleased to pick up an abnormality on physical examination. Basically it comes down to the fact that doctors like to be problem solvers and therefore it would be disingenuous to pretend there is no self-satisfaction upon finding, when examining a patient, those things that you had deduced from an interview would likely be present.

Lymph gland enlargement is termed:

1. lymphogranuloma venereum
2. lymphadenitis
3. lymphadenopathy
4. lymphing

Answer: 3. From lympha which is Latin meaning "clear spring water" and pathos which is Greek for "suffering."

Lymph gland enlargement may signify:

1. infectious mononucleosis
2. lymph gland cancer
3. leukemia
4. all of the above

Answer: 4. That was a giveaway. If you are a teenager and have swollen lymph glands, a fever, feel worn out, and find out that your girl or boyfriend feels the same way, then there is a strong likelihood that you have mono (infectious mononucleosis). Many other causes of enlarged glands do exist, however, including lymph gland tumours and leukemias.

Now even if it is exciting to pick up a finding on examining a patient, you've got to have the good sense to not let the patient know it. Most doctors realize that. Most, but not all. I once brought my then infant son into an out-of-town emergency department after he had developed a high fever. The physician examining him was looking very intently at some marks on his skin. Marks that had been there since birth and obviously had nothing to do with the fever. "Hmm, look at this," he said. "And this also. Hmm. Hmm." The doctor became increasingly ebullient. He was so excited I thought he was going to burst. "Yes, yes; I think he may have von Recklinghausen's" *You putz,* I thought. *Don't you have at least half a brain. Here you are telling me some devastating news and you look thrilled about it.* Well, as it turns out my son did not have that rare disease of nerve tumour formation. *So screw you,* I thought (and would have loved to have said, but didn't).

I left the room whilst Mr. Ferguson got dressed then I re-entered and sat down on a chair directly in front of him. I explained to Mr. Ferguson that he had some worrisome findings. His fatigue was certainly non-specific but given his having night sweats and lymph gland enlargement we had to pursue things further.

I always have my office patients get dressed and then seated directly in front of me before I talk to them about my conclusions. Even at the best of times people are uncomfortable when seeing a doctor. Add to that their concerns that they have something seriously wrong and what is certainly not needed on this less-than-level playing field is to have the patient sitting there almost naked confronting a fully clothed physician sitting professorially behind a large desk. It's also worth noting that studies have found that patients' recollections of the length of time that the doctor spoke with them is greatly influenced by whether the doctor was sitting or standing during the discussion. If the doctor was standing the patients significantly underestimated the duration of their meeting. No doubt the patient got the impression the doctor was in a rush. Truth of the matter is, doctors are always in a rush. But if you don't want to make it transparent to the patient, then you make sure you are sitting while you are talking to them.

How to preserve a patient's dignity is something that gets taught with varying degrees of success in medical school. Some professors are the best of role models. And then there are some like a former department head of a university teaching hospital where I spent some time.

One day, this particular physician and his house-staff (interns and residents; of which I was one) were circled around a patient's bedside. The patient was a thirty-four-year-old woman in hospital for investigation of possible liver disease. The staff physician, a middle-aged man by the name of Michael Deans, was describing the physical examination findings seen with liver disease. In order to illustrate his point, Dr. Deans pulled the sheets off the patient. It was obvious that it had never occurred to him to ask her permission or to warn her. It was equally obvious that she was entirely naked and that Dr. Deans thought that to be all the better to illustrate the physical exam findings.

Being a junior physician I stood silently and felt helpless. If I did as instinct and morality dictated and pulled this woman's sheets back up I knew I would get Dr. Deans thoroughly ticked off. You don't want to do that to the physician who will be giving you your evaluation. I looked at my assembled colleagues. We were all shifting in discomfort. No one did anything.

I looked back at the patient. She was obviously embarrassed, but she too did nothing. Lying there in bed, worried you have some God-awful illness, thinking that the learned professor is the one who is going to save your life, the last thing in the world that you want to do is risk offending your white-jacketed saviour. As doctors we are seeing people at their most vulnerable. And vulnerable people will put up with a lot of crap. So she lay still.

I started to think about the long line of historical villains whose crime was passivity when action had been called for. I had to do something. I couldn't let this poor woman lie there naked with ten people standing around her as if she was a steer up for auction. As I was trying to summon up my courage a fellow resident of obviously greater fortitude reached over to the foot of the bed and pulled the sheets up. Dr. Deans glowered and pulled them back down. The resident pulled them up again. Down. Up. A power struggle. After this tug of war had gone on for what felt like an eternity (but was, no doubt, just a few seconds), Dr. Deans turned around and walked out of the room. We did not follow. Our evaluations were not great. And I did not care. Sort of. Next time, I decided, I would be the one to respond first. Thankfully, the situation did not arise again. So I can feel righteous that I really, truly was planning on doing "the right thing" should it happen again; it just didn't happen to.

When I sat down with Mr. Ferguson I went through the old dilemma of how much information would be the right amount to impart in such a circumstance. Though I had been taught it in medical school, it was only after I was in clinical practice that I realized the degree of truth in the notion that once you have told a patient that they have something seriously wrong, they retain little you say thereafter. I used to get frustrated when, despite having given a patient a detailed explanation of the illness that they were suffering from, I would be told at a subsequent meeting that I had not let them know such and such or when I would get a call from a frantic relative wondering "just what *is* wrong" with so and so. It was only with time that I came to realize that people turned off once they heard the mention of cancer or other such horrific disease.

It took a while to learn to simply explain the basics, let the patient mull that over, and then wait for questions. Answers can be given with detail commensurate with the questions asked. Does this approach work for everyone? Of course not. Some people prefer to hear everything, others just the bare minimum. The difficulty is in predicting who wants to hear what.

Mr. Ferguson went on to have further testing and ultimately a diagnosis of Hodgkin's Disease was made. Fortunately, it responded well to treatment and he went into remission. A sigh of relief. His and mine. And crossed fingers that it will not recur.

Mrs. Woods and Mr. Ferguson had both come to see me for what they described as tiredness yet the causes were light years apart. You have to keep an open mind. You never know what might be lurking behind a seemingly innocuous complaint.

Chapter Two

CHEST PAIN, NEEDLESS TESTS, AND WHAT
THEY DON'T TEACH YOU AT HARVARD
MEDICAL SCHOOL

He was scared. Terrified in fact. And who could blame him? John's father had died suddenly from a heart attack when John was just a child of eight. And now that John himself was the father of a young child, it was no wonder that he was frightened when he started getting chest pains. He first noticed them when he was walking up a hill at the golf course. "A dull pressure right here," he told me, putting a fist over the left side of his chest.

John has a textbook case of:

1. spasm of the swallowing tube (esophageal spasm)
2. angina
3. chest wall strain
4. a bruised rib

Answer: 2. If you got this one correct I am afraid you don't go to the head of the class. There's no room there, for everyone has likely got this one right, unless of course they are not familiar with the term angina.

Angina is:

1. a Rolling Stones' hit
2. chest pain due to heart disease
3. a sore throat

Answer: 2. Give yourself two bonus marks if you also guessed 3. Ninety-nine percent of the time "angina'" is used as a synonym for "angina pectoris," which in turn means chest pain due to coronary artery disease. Coronary artery disease is the condition of narrowing of those arteries which feed the heart with blood (and hence oxygen). Nonetheless, there are other forms of angina which have nothing to do with the heart. One such form is a sore throat.

Most all physicians would (and should!) quickly realize what John's chest pains represent and would pursue things accordingly.

Many people however do not present to their doctor with typical chest pain. And medical scholars, in uncharacteristically simple and clear language, have termed this lack of typical pain "atypical chest pain." I can tell you that I see a heck of a lot more patients with so-called "atypical" chest pain than with "typical" chest pain. Unfortunately, in medical school, whereas the professors spend umpteen hours teaching about the classical chest pain of angina, they don't teach much about atypical chest pain.

Let's say you have generally been healthy. Your parents are well into their sixties without major health problems and you don't suffer from hypertension, diabetes, or high cholesterol. Suddenly you start having chest pains. They first began when you were walking down the street. A stabbing pain, like a knife. It "went right through" you and as my patients often say, it was "right in the heart." It lasted a second or two, went away for a moment then came back. That went on for a few minutes following which you were okay again. Except that you were worried that it might be a heart problem. So you went to see your doctor who gave you the low down.

And the low down is that your pains are caused by:

1. a heart condition (boy, I wish I knew what that meant)
2. anxiety attacks
3. a hiatus hernia
4. any of the above
5. none of the above

Answer: 5. So then, what is the low down? Well, what you really needed was a good dose of reassurance and little else. The pain you were having was almost certainly just the harmless (though admittedly painful) spasm of muscles between the ribs (the intercostal muscles). With few exceptions you should be told that there is nothing to worry about, the pain will likely come and go a few times then ultimately subside and you should just live with it until then.

Now, maybe that is what you should be told but in reality what often happens is that before any diagnosis is arrived at you will be sent for an EKG, some blood tests, a urine sample, and more likely than not, an exercise stress test (wherein your heart is monitored whilst you exercise on a treadmill). Why, you might ask, would your doctor order these studies if they are not necessary? There are a number of possible reasons.

Firstly, your doctor may simply not be familiar with this form of chest pain and is using the shotgun approach (that is, fire your tests in all directions and you'll probably hit the right diagnosis somewhere). Alternatively, your doctor may have the "I don't want to get burned approach." Not so very long ago a doctor's main apprehension in missing a diagnosis was simply that he or she did not want to let the patient down. Nowadays, however, with the proliferation of malpractice suits there has been a major shift in a doctor's rationale for doing things. "Covering your ass" has become the motto of the day. Regrettably. Perhaps inevitably.

"Overinvestigating" also arises from patient expectations. When a physician senses that a patient equates the degree of thoroughness with the quantity of tests performed, it should be no surprise that physicians feel compelled to meet these expectations. More than once I have heard patients, in reference to their doctors, state that "my doctor is very thorough; you wouldn't believe the number of tests he put me through." And lo and behold "thank God, nothing serious was found." But this was virtually a foregone conclusion. If there is a low probability of a test being abnormal it should not be a surprise when it turns out normal. "Yes," you say, "but what if it ended up showing something." Well, if it does then there is a strong likelihood the result is abnormal but you are not. A "false positive." And this happens because tests are fallible. And when the test result comes up abnormal, what then? Well, that leads to further tests and then more tests and then ... well, you get the point. The initial symptom by then has probably gone away, but by then the system is on a roll and you are rolling with it.

Many patients and physicians alike simply do not recognize a test's limitations. Let us say that you have chest pain and your doctor sends you for a "stress test." This typically involves walking on a treadmill for ten minutes or so during which time your EKG is monitored. If it becomes abnormal a diagnosis of heart disease is made. If it is normal reassurance is given. Nice and simple. Too simple. There is a very high rate of inaccuracy with this test. Indeed someone can have severe blockages in their coronary arteries, but still have a normal test. I've seen several patients who had a normal test only to then go on to have a heart attack within days. One patient within hours. Conversely I have seen many, many patients with very abnormal results on a stress test who had no heart disease at all. The bottom line is: no test is perfect. The corollary therefore must be: why is my doctor sending me for a test which might be more misleading than helpful? Good question. Remember to ask your doctor. But I'll tell you now anyhow. The test often *is* accurate *if* you have typical symptoms. If you ain't got typical symptoms then the likelihood of a false result is much higher. So to routinely screen everybody, in particular those without symptoms, is often a bad idea. But many doctors just don't know it.

There is another major reason a doctor might order some studies even when they may not be indicated. As much as I hate to admit it, it is not unusual for a quite cozy relationship to exist between the physician ordering a test and the physician getting paid for supervising and interpreting the test. The reason for this is not difficult to fathom. They are often the same person. Even if the doctor does not in any way honestly feel that is the reason they've ordered something, once there is a financial benefit, can impartiality be guaranteed? For example, let's say that a cardiologist (hey, I'm not a cardiologist so they are fair game) sees you because you're having chest pain. If all he (or she of course) performs is a consultation (in which you are interviewed and examined and a letter is then sent to your family doctor) the cardiologist would get paid about one hundred dollars. At least in Canada. In the U.S. you could triple (or more) this. But, and this is a big but, if you need further tests (and few cardiologists decide you don't) then let's tally the score (oh, and by the way I am not including the charge for the lab's equipment and supplies, just the direct fee to the doctor for interpreting the test):

1) consultation	$100.00
2) exercise stress test	$50.00
3) portable heart monitor	$50.00
4) thalium stress test	$75.00
5) MUGA scan	$75.00
6) angiogram	$300.00
Total:	$650.00

So, a $100 consultation is turned into a $650 consultation. Did you need all those tests? Maybe you did, and, maybe you didn't. Knew I should have gone into cardiology. Damn.

Now I don't want to sound overly sanctimonious here. I too send patients for tests that I then interpret and get paid for. Not many, but some. And I have to ask myself each time, does this patient really need this test? Is it possible that financial gain is influencing my decision? I try hard to be sure that I am ordering the tests only for the purest of reasons. But can I ever be completely certain? Well, being the moral, upstanding citizen that I am, of course I can be certain. I think.

How about something as simple as the need for return visits. Let's say you have high blood pressure. Not terrible; just higher than it should be. Your doctor asks you to come back every two months to have it re-checked. Or perhaps to come every month. Or maybe even biweekly. Which schedule is best? And how are you to know? Could it be that the optimal frequency of follow-up visits depends as much or more on how busy the doctor is rather than on how much of a problem your blood pressure is? Could be. Sometimes is.

Another thing about lab tests. It is very common practice to tell patients that they will be called only if their lab results come back abnormal. Like the old adage goes, "no news is good news." Well I've got some news of my own: when it comes to your health the only certain thing about no news is that it is no news. You should never, ever assume that no news is good news. Want to know why? Thought you'd never ask.

Let's trace the sequence of events when, for example, you have a blood test:

step one:	the lab requisition is filled out.
step two:	the lab requisition is given to the patient.
step three:	the lab takes the blood sample.
step four:	the lab processes the sample.
step five:	the lab sends the report to the doctor.
step six:	the secretary puts the report out for the doctor to review it.
step seven:	the doctor signs off the report giving the secretary instructions as to what follow-up arrangements should be made for the patient whose results are abnormal.
step eight:	the secretary arranges the appropriate follow-up.
step nine:	the patient attends the scheduled follow-up appointment.

Now lets look at what not only can, but often does happen:

step one:	the doctor forgets to sign the requisition so the test doesn't get done.

<u>step two:</u>	the patient loses the requisition and forgets that some (perhaps crucial) tests had been ordered.
<u>step three:</u>	the lab overlooks one of the ticks on the requisition and thus an ordered test fails to get done.
<u>step four:</u>	the lab loses the sample.
<u>step five:</u>	the lab fails to send the report to the doctor or it gets lost in the mail or it goes to the wrong doctor. (My associate [a.k.a. my wife] has the same name as three other doctors in the region; you can guess how often she gets results on patients she has never heard of.)
<u>step six:</u>	the secretary puts out a stack of lab results for the doctor's review, but fails to notice that one of the pieces of paper has fallen into the garbage pail.
<u>step seven:</u>	the doctor writes instructions for the secretary, but the scrawl is largely illegible and thus,
<u>step eight:</u>	she misinterprets the scrawl and hence, fails to make the requested follow-up appointment and
<u>step nine:</u>	the doctor does not have a fail-safe mechanism by which any of the above errors would be caught.

So-o-o-o, if you assume that your lab results must be normal since you never got a call back from your doctor then you are putting absolutely incredible faith in a system fraught with shortcomings. In which case I would strongly recommend that you avoid door-to-door salespeople, certain southern Florida realtors, and re-runs of the PTL Club.

Patricia White, a forty-eight-year-old woman, was referred because she was having chest pain. It was a burning discomfort in the area of the breast-bone (the sternum).

"Well, doctor," she explained, "it comes on after I eat and takes about an hour or so to go away." She paused. I remained silent (the golden rule of history taking; "let the patient do the talking"). She noticed my expectant expression and elaborated. "I find I can get it to settle down if I take some Maalox."

"Aha," I thought to myself, she has solved the issue without my saying a word. Burning chest pain, after meals, in sternal area, resolves with antacid ...

The diagnosis must be:

1. angina (clue: if you guessed this then you're not paying attention)
2. a hiatus hernia
3. inflamation in the outermost lining of the heart ("pericarditis")

4. gastro-esophageal reflux (the coming up of some stomach acid into the esophagus).

Answer: 4. But if you guessed 2 instead then you get half marks since you may or may not be right. People can get gastro-esophageal reflux whether or not they have a hiatus hernia. I can also tell you that many, many people go around thinking they have an illness because an x-ray showed a hiatus hernia. But up to 50 percent of healthy adults have hiatus hernias found on x-ray and the bulk of these patients do not have symptoms referable to them. In other words, a hiatus hernia is often an incidental, clinically insignificant problem. But some doctors do not realize this and ascribe some nonspecific, somewhat nebulous symptoms to what is actually an insignificant radiological finding and forevermore patients will go around blaming their stomach upset "on that damn hernia of mine." Doctors who know better will still often label a patient's vague stomach complaints on a minimal hiatus hernia showing up on x-ray. Why? Because people like a label. Doctors and patients alike. Also, it can take a lot longer to sit down with a patient and explain why the diagnosis is uncertain rather than giving a quick label, maybe an equally quick prescription and getting on to the next patient

There are some cardinal rules of history taking that all medical students are taught. Sort of the medical version of the journalist's who, what, where, when, and why. As med students it is drilled into us to establish what brings a symptom on, what makes it worse, and what makes it better. If we can get the patient to volunteer this information, all the better. Otherwise, you can end up putting words into your patient's mouth that end up simply misleading you ...

"So, Mr. Smith I see you're here to see me because of chest pain."
"Uhuh."
"Is it kind of a heavy pain?"
"Well, I guess so."
"I see. And does it go away in just a couple of minutes?"
"Well, sort of."
"And do you feel short of breath when it happens?"
"Yeah, maybe a little bit."
"I see. Could be angina. I'll book you for some tests. In the meantime, why don't you start taking these nitroglycerin pills."
End of conversation.

I admit to some (but not a lot) exaggeration in the above scenario. Oh, and believe me, this does happen. Often. No, not my exaggeration.

Physicians, like an overly aggressive lawyer, leading the client. But in the examining room there is no opposing attorney to shout "objection, your honour."

Client. Yuk. That's the new catchword in health care circles. *Client*. This is meant to *empower* the individual. Give me a break. A letter in the Candian Medical Association Journal aptly states the case: "Doctors treat patients; clients are found in lawyers' offices and brothels."

The other new catchword to describe patients is *consumer* as in "Mr. Jacobs is a consumer of health care." Damn patients will eat you alive, I guess.

Acting as a consultant, I occasionally will see a patient who, in the middle (or sometimes even earlier) of my history taking will express indignation that I do not already have their answers as recorded by their family practitioner. They consider it offensive that I should have to ask them what they feel are redundant questions. Indeed, it is quite true that many of the questions have previously been asked. Nonetheless, asking them again is almost always a necessity. This is because obtaining a history is a very subjective process. It is not the same as having someone fill out a blank questionnaire. Thankfully. It surely would make medicine a bore if the individual doctor's skills were of no consequence. Each physician comes to rely on the history that they have obtained to be the valid one. The corollary of course is that not all physicians can be right if they get different histories from the same patient. Any wonder why medicine is less than a precise science?

Mrs. Sandy Watson was a forty-five-year-old woman sent to see me with "chest pain — rule out angina." And indeed her story did sound suspicious for a heart problem in that she complained of a pain in the left side of her chest. But, unlike typical angina, her pain was primarily an ache rather than a pressure. And it would start in the back and then travel around to the front. Basic investigations were normal. I reassured her that it was not her heart, but I felt uncomfortable not knowing more definitively what, in fact, it was. Well, two days later it became clear. She had broken out with a band-like series of blisters over her chest in precisely the area that her pain had been.

She had:

1. shingles
2. AIDS
3. a yeast infection
4. dermatitis herpetiformis

Answer: 1. Shingles is the rash that occurs when a long dormant chicken pox virus (varicella zoster) reactivates. When it does it typically erupts along the length and breadth of a nerve that supplies sensation to a part of the body (a "dermatome").

One of my all time favourites when it comes to disease names is the condition going by the wonderful moniker of Tietse's syndrome.

Tietse's syndrome is named after:

1. an African fruit fly
2. a South American parasite
3. a teeny town in Tanzania
4. Alexander Tietze.

Answer: 4. Yes indeed; it was for a German surgeon living 1864–1927 that this syndrome was named.

If you are suffering from Tietse's syndrome you would have an annoying pain in:

1. the region between the shoulder blades
2. the perineum (the area between the anus and the genitals)
3. the big toe
4. one of the costo-chondral joints (the area where the ribs meet the breastbone).

Answer: 4. The cause of this condition? Unknown. The treatment? Symptomatic. The prognosis? Excellent. By the way, this condition is to be differentiated from African Sleeping Sickness caused by the Tsetse fly.

A number of years ago a woman in her early twenties presented to an emergency department with complaints of vague breathlessness and a bit of chest discomfort. Gail was fully assessed, was thought to be suffering from anxiety and she was sent on her way. Her symptoms recurred and she went back to the emergency. Again, nothing untoward was found and she was discharged home. A few days later she yet again felt chest pain and returned to the hospital. For the third time no significant problem was identified and she was reassured and discharged. Five hours later she went into shock and died.

A young woman with breathlessness and chest pain who then suddenly goes into shock is probably suffering from:

1. a blood clot in the lung

2. a perforated ulcer
3. an anxiety attack
4. a gallbladder attack

Answer: 1.

An autopsy revealed a massive pulmonary embolism. That is, a blood clot that has travelled from a distant vein to the artery that goes to the lungs (the pulmonary artery). This type of blood clot typically forms in the deep veins of the legs (a condition termed thrombophlebitis or, for short, phlebitis) in patients who are bedbound, such as when recovering from surgery. It also occurs in patients who are "hypercoagulable," which is to say their blood is overly prone to clotting.

Why might a young woman be prone to blood clotting?

1. if there is a family history of clotting disorders
2. if she is a smoker
3. if she is on the birth control pill
4. if she is overweight
5. all of the above

Answer: 5. Although the pill is taken uneventfully by millions upon millions of woman, there are some perfectly healthy woman who run into disastrous complications. Gail was one of them.

Pulmonary embolism is a diagnosis that haunts doctors. And it is precisely because of people like Gail. People can seem perfectly healthy except for some seemingly innocuous, nonspecific complaints. And then suddenly they die.

The risks entailed by taking oral contraceptives have been carefully documented by epidemiologists (physicians who study patterns of disease). What has not been looked at, however, is the much greater incidence of psychological and physiological morbidity caused by problems that are only *indirectly* attributable to being on the pill. Let me illustrate.

Barbara was thirty years of age and had been on oral contraceptives for three years. She was in generally excellent health. One day she developed some fairly mild chest pain; mild enough that were she not on the pill she would have ignored it. However, knowing that the pill can cause serious side effects, she went to the hospital to have things checked out. She left work early (her boss none too pleased), arranged baby-sitting as she knew she would be late getting home, and she drove to the hospital. After waiting the requisite eternity in the emergency department she got seen by a doctor who, given that Barbara was on the pill, was understandably concerned about her symptoms and felt that further tests should be done.

Mandatory tests for a patient such as this should include all of the following *except*:

1. a chest x-ray
2. a urine sample
3. an EKG (electrocardiogram; also goes by the alias ECG)
4. a blood oxygen measurement

Answer: 2.

To obtain a measurement of the blood oxygen level one must have a needle inserted into an artery. This is:

1. true
2. false

Answer: 2. Traditionally we have done what is known as arterial blood gas samples ("ABGs"), however we can now use a probe (placed on a finger or an ear lobe) which is quite reliable at giving oxygen level measurements ("oximetry").

Arterial blood gas measurements are:

1. a big deal
2. no big deal

Answer: 1. They hurt like hell. The test involves putting a needle into the (radial) artery in the wrist. Unlike a vein, the artery is deep to the skin and can only be felt, not seen. The needle has to go in a fair way and into a sensitive area. All in all, a very bad experience. But sometimes it really is necessary since an oximetry probe measurement is not always reliable.

Why do we doctors have the unerring habit of telling patients that a test is "not that bad" when it is "that bad?" It'll hurt "just a bit" we say when it is likely to hurt "just a bit" only if you just happen to be lucky enough to be in a deep coma at the time. Well, underplaying the degree of discomfort (okay, okay, let's call a spade a spade; it's not discomfort we're talking about, it's pain pure and simple) does serve at least one function: it's easier to get the patient to agree to the test.

After the basic studies were done it was still unclear if Barbara's chest pain was or was not due to a pulmonary embolism. Accordingly, it was concluded that she needed a lung scan. This is a test wherein a small dose of radioactive material is injected into a vein and another dose is inhaled. It is often, but not always, an exceptionally helpful way of sorting out if a pulmonary embolism is or is not present. Problem was, there was no way of getting it done in the middle of the night and thus Barbara had to wait overnight in the emergency department on a stretcher. As well, in case she did have a clot, she had to be treated immediately, even without a definite diagnosis, since it would be too dangerous to delay therapy. Accordingly she had an intravenous started and was given blood thinners. The potential risk of hemorrhaging resultant from blood thinners was explained to her. Brain and stomach bleeding from blood thinners are not just theoretical events. They happen.

Of course, with the lung scan not being done until the next morning and not being reported until that afternoon, she had to miss work that day.

Around 4 p.m., long after her original symptoms had passed, the lung scan was reported as normal. The doctor reassured Barbara and she was discharged home. All was well.

Except that the patient had been worried sick that something life-threatening might be present, she had missed a day and a half of work, she had not slept and was exhausted, she had had a number of painful procedures, she had been exposed to radiation and to the risks of being on a blood thinner, and the cost to the health care system was several thousand dollars. And all for a disease which she turned out not to have. Yet each and every thing that was done was appropriate.

And you know what? Nowhere will you find this type of morbidity reported. No study will detail just how many thousands of patients just like Barbara exist. Patients who undergo mental, physical, and financial suffering not because of a dangerous complication of being on the pill; but rather because of the quite justified perception that there *might* be a problem.

Chapter Three

HEADACHES, CARING FOR COLLEAGUES, AND
SLEEPING WITH PATIENTS

Margaret was a pleasant fifty-year-old woman who did not like to complain but, on the prompting of her daughter, she decided that she probably should see somebody about the headaches she had recently developed.

She described them as being "vice-like." They were made worse by lying down and improved when she was standing. They were associated with nausea and vomiting.

This would seem to be relatively sparse information with which to establish any sort of diagnosis yet in fact this information gave considerable insight into what was likely going on.

Margaret was most likely suffering from:

1. tension headaches
2. migraines
3. a brain tumour
4. a brain aneurism

Answer: 3.

The clues pointing toward a diagnosis of brain tumour were as follows:

i) *The headaches were new.* When someone who virtually never gets headaches suddenly develops them that is definitely a worrisome sign. Relatively "benign" headache disorders (like migraine and tension headaches) are generally chronic problems whereas headaches due to something catastrophic (such as a brain tumour) are something the patient almost always recognizes as being decidedly new and different for them.

   Tension headaches. Oh, how I hate that term. Does it mean that the patient is tense or that the scalp muscles are tense? I don't know. Neither does anyone else. Seeing as medical science has not proved the latter to actually occur in this condition I suspect the ambiguity is intentional. Most people recognize their tension headaches when they have them, realize they will go away within hours, and treat them symptomatically with plain analgesics. Margaret, however, had a headache the likes of which she had never before experienced. Hence, a warning to me that her headaches might not be the run-of-the-mill type.

ii) *The headaches were like a vice.* This is typical of headaches of the "tension" variety but can also be seen with headaches due to brain tumours.

iii) *The headaches were made worse by lying down.* A key point. Tension headaches are generally minimized if one lies down. Migraine headaches also tend to be improved by lying down. Conversely, headaches due to a source of increased pressure within the brain itself ("raised intra-cranial pressure"), such as commonly occurs if one has a brain tumour, are worsened when supine.

iv) *The headaches were associated with nausea and vomiting.* This could occur with a variety of types of headache. Nevertheless, raised intra-cranial pressure typically causes nausea and vomiting and thus this feature has to be taken very seriously.

Having come to a preliminary diagnosis within minutes of meeting Margaret, the tendency would be to immediately order the definitive test.

The single best test for determining if someone has a brain tumour is a:

1. C.A.T. (computerized axial tomography) scan
2. M.R.I. (magnetic resonance imaging) scan

Answer: 2. If you answered 1 you get one-half marks since in most institutions C.A.T. scanners are much more likely to be accessible than are the more costly M.R.I. scanners. (Of interest, magnetic resonance imaging used to be termed "nuclear magnetic resonance" until the powers that be decided that people would not understand that not everything nuclear was synonymous with horrific).

Frequently I will be referred patients with headaches who have had neither of the two tests listed above. Not that the tests were not necessary. Rather, they were *not available*. Instead, these patients have had second-rate investigations like skull x-rays and nuclear isotope brain scans that are generally quite useless. Why are the better tests not the ones being done? Simple answer to that one. Money. Pure and simple. Health care facilities know that restricting the availability of certain state-of-the-art tests translates into saving dollars. The net result is that family doctors are often *not even allowed* to order C.A.T. scans, never mind M.R.I. scans. Hell, if I was the patient I would want the most accurate and safest test and I would want it NOW. I wonder how many health care administrators have skull x-rays when what they really need is a C.A.T. scan.

Now I guess I should get down off my soap-box (or high horse, as the case may be) and be fair to hospital administrators, up here north of the forty-ninth, for there *are* substantial abuses of the available technologies. Many people with headaches who need nothing more than reassurance get sent off for further investigation primarily because physicians are afraid of missing things. And that is especially true if we are looking after patients who happen to be doctors or doctors' relatives.

God, I would feel dreadful if I overlooked a diagnosis on one of my colleagues. So, I admit it; when I have a doctor as a patient I too send them for more tests than are absolutely necessary. And I see them urgently even for non-urgent problems. Even if that means other less well-connected patients wait longer to get into the office. Do I feel guilty about this? Sure. But I have my guilty conscience eased somewhat when I hear that my friend, the one who gets caught in radar traps more frequently than a Manhattan hooker turns tricks, has not had a traffic ticket in five years. He's a cop. And please understand that when doctors and their families get sent for umpteen tests that you wouldn't get routinely, that most definitely does *not* mean they are getting better medical care. More care, yes. Faster care, yes. Better care, no. In fact when it comes to doctors and their tests, less is often best. Remember what I said in an earlier chapter about the inaccuracy rate of tests and the system pushing you along once you're on board? Well, that holds especially true for doctors when they are patients; that is, they get over-investigated and hence are more likely to have falsely abnormal tests turn up which leads to more investigations and more of this and more of that and on it goes.

Another way in which doctors are short-changed when it comes to their own health care is the flippant way in which advice is often obtained. Physicians are notorious for getting "corridor consults." That is, when they are feeling unwell, they will mention their symptoms to a colleague in the corridor of the hospital. A quick diagnosis is made and treatment rapidly started. No full history. No examination. In other words, what even the worst of doctors would not do to their patients, the best of doctors does to one's colleagues. I know of more than one physician that has died because of this. One case was that of a doctor who was given a corridor consult and quickly diagnosed as having chest pains due to acid indigestion. The next day he died of a heart attack. So I adamantly refuse to give colleagues advice unless they first come into the office and go through the same rigmarole that the rest of my patients go through. Sometimes they get ticked off by this. But, I hold my ground. I know I am right. And I savour that feeling — knowing with absolute certainty that this is one of those exceedingly rare issues for which I can be entitled to self-righteous satisfaction in standing by a principle.

Back to Margaret. Though a case could be made to go directly to a C.A.T. or M.R.I. scan, in reality few physicians would do so without first examining the patient. Indeed, if a doctor by-passes the exam altogether you might just think twice about what kind of doctor you have. The physical examination often gives additional clues which might both corroborate the working diagnosis (that is, what you suspect is wrong based on the history) and could turn up additional important clinical features which would be missed otherwise. For instance, perhaps Margaret's headache was simply due to high blood pressure.

High blood pressure is a common cause of headache. This is:

1. true
2. false

Answer: 2. High blood pressure rarely causes headaches. When it does it is generally only if the blood pressure is very, very high.

I checked Margaret's blood pressure and found it to be normal. I then checked her pulse. If fast it could signify possible thyroid over-activity or excess levels of adrenaline.

A normal pulse rate is:

1. 60 to 100
2. 70 to 80
3. 50 to 90

Answer: 1. Note that one's pulse rate is not a static thing, but in fact constantly varies. No one's pulse is always 70. Well, there are exceptions to that — if you have a permanent pace-maker (though nowadays they sometimes use variable rate pace-makers, but let's not confuse the issue).

The pulse is measured by:

1. counting each beat for six seconds and multiplying by ten
2. counting each beat for fifteen seconds and multiplying by four
3. counting each beat for thirty seconds and multiplying by two
4. all of the above

Answer: 4. The pulse rate is simply the number of pulses (that is, heart beats) per minute. That seems so straightforward, but obviously it is not seeing as I find that very few people actually know how to measure it. The simplest way is to just count each beat for an entire minute — if there are sixty beats in a minute then your pulse is sixty per minute. Because it's too time consuming to count for a whole minute, most doctors just count the number of beats in six seconds and multiply by ten.

Margaret's pulse rate was normal.

The next thing I did was to carefully examine Margaret's eyes, for this gives key information about an entire nerve pathway. Like an electrical circuit, one interruption and the whole system fails. In this case the circuit begins with light hitting the back of the eye (the "retina") which then triggers nerve impulses which course through to the brain. Return impulses cause the pupils to narrow ("constrict") in response to light.

I checked to see if Margaret's pupils were of similar size. I looked to see if shining a light in *one* eye caused *both* pupils to constrict as it should. Visual fields were assessed by noting if Margaret could recognize my fingers moving in front of her. All checked out fine.

Next, I took out my ophthalmoscope so that I could peer right to the back of Margaret's eyes. This is truly one of those intriguing things that just can't be understood unless you can do it yourself. People often feel that you must be looking directly into the brain if not necessarily into the soul (to wax poetic). Regrettably, it is quite a bit more mundane than that. The ophthalmoscope allows one to see through to the back of the eye where the retina is located. Therein we see a fine network of blood vessels emanating from a central hub called the *optic disc*. Just imagine looking at the bottom of an uprooted tree with its roots radiating out in all directions.

As I looked through the ophthalmoscope into Margaret's eyes I paused. Was I really seeing what I thought I was? I stepped back to rest for a moment. Picking up the instrument I peered again. There was no doubt about the diagnosis now. Poor Margaret.

A brain tumour can lead to elevated pressure within the brain. This pressure cannot be transmitted in many directions as of course the brain is encased in a rigid skull. Because there is a communication between the brain and the orbits (the "eyeballs"), a build-up of pressure within the brain can be transmitted to the retina where, on ophthalmoscopic examination, swelling of the optic disc can be identified. This is termed *papilledema*. And it is of unparalleled importance. Its presence signifies an impending catastrophe.

Margaret had papilledema. A subsequent C.A.T. scan confirmed the presence of a brain tumour.

I well remember reading the subsequent operative report. It didn't seem to make sense. The operation had begun at 08:00 hours yet finished at 10:00 hours. But the note indicated they had been able to entirely remove Margaret's brain tumour. I read the report again and again. Then it became clear. The operation had not been two hours long. It had been twenty-six hours long. Ever since then I have not begrudged my neurosurgery colleagues their substantial incomes. Well, maybe I've begrudged a bit.

When assessing someone for the problem of headache a physician generally will do a full neurological examination. This is:

1. true
2. false
3. sort of true

Answer: 3. Sort of true. Score equal marks if you chose option 2. As one of my former professors once said in a moment of candour, "no one ever does a full neurological examination — it would take too long." Which reminds me of the jargon we typically used when as residents (doctors

doing specialty training) we would note in our reports "CNS — NAD."
This means "central neurological system — no abnormality detected."
At least in theory that's what it means. In practice we all knew that it
really stood for "central neurological system — not actually done." Too
time consuming.

I find that patients are often surprised that you would want to examine
any part of them other than where their apparent symptom is. If Karen
has a headache, why in the world, she might wonder, would I want to
examine her abdomen. Bill might wonder the same thing, but in
general it is more of an issue if the patient is female and the doctor is
male. I imagine it was not much of a concern years ago, but now that
the press is replete with cases of doctors' sexual impropriety it certainly
is something that doctors and patients think about. Lots.

A very tricky problem this. If I pre-emptively explain to Karen the
rationale for doing a full exam (which is indeed necessary; headaches
could be due to metastatic breast cancer for example), this may suggest
that there is something I'm about to do which might otherwise be
misconstrued as being improper. It also suggests that there may be some
underlying mistrust. As well, it would then require a discussion about the
many possible things I would look for during an examination and such a
conversation would not only be immensely time consuming, but would
raise worries where none should have existed.

On the other hand, if I offer no explanation maybe Karen will think
I'm one of those deviant doctors she reads about in the papers. Can't
win, eh? In any event, what I generally do is simply say that I would like
to examine them and explain why only if they ask.

Even seemingly innocent things now have the potential, given the
right circumstances, to take on sexual overtones and this can make
things terribly awkward. I'll give you some examples.

When I check someone's blood pressure I make sure, as does
virtually every other physician, that I am beside the patient's legs, never
between them. When checking a patient's eyes with an ophthalmoscope
not only do I ensure I am beside the patient's legs (at times making you
into a contortionist worthy of the Cirque du Soleil), but you have to
make sure the room's lighting is just right. Too dark and some patient or
other will think you are up to no good. Too bright and you simply can't
get a good look into the eyes.

Sometimes, I think despairingly, this has all gone too far.

For years I have kept my patients still when I listen to their
lungs by placing my right hand on their right shoulder. No big deal.
Now I wonder if they think I'm being sexually inappropriate; too
much touching, you know. I was taught to put a hand on the
patient's forehead when doing an ophthalmologic exam so that I

don't accidentally bang into their eye with the instrument. Now I think twice. And as I examine some women I can't help but wonder if they are asking themselves if I am spending a bit too long examining their breasts or their abdomens or ...

One young woman always comes into the office and greets me with "how ya doin' handsome." Forgetting that she clearly has more need of an ophthalmologist than of an internist, that greeting now gives me chills. Maybe it's not just a friendly, harmless salutation. Maybe it has sexual overtones. Should I say something to her? Or will that just bewilder her and make an asexual greeting into something different?

Recently I bumped into a former patient in a busy shopping centre. I had looked after her diabetes during a complicated but ultimately very successful pregnancy. "Doctor Blumer!" she shouted, having spied me from across the concourse. She ran to where I stood. "Remember me? I want to thank you again for all you did." Sounds benign enough, does it not? Except that she was giving me a bear hug and a kiss as she said this. I thanked her for her thanks, put my head down and hoped that my bald spot made me blend in with the ceramic floor. And all the while I kept thinking, "will people think I slept with this woman? Will they report me to the College of Physicians and Surgeons?" And then I got mad. Hell, why do I have to feel guilty that a woman has embraced me out of thanks for helping her have a healthy child? What in the world has the practice of medicine come to? Maybe things have gone just a bit too far. Like by several light years. Or maybe I worry too much. Or maybe not.

You'd figure that of all male physicians (sexual misconduct accusations against female doctors being almost unheard of), gynecologists would be at the highest risk of being charged with sexual impropriety. I certainly figured that. I was wrong. As a gynecologist colleague of mine said, "when a woman sees me she knows and the courts would know what is going to happen." An internal exam is obviously part of normal routine. It is when a woman sees a family doctor because of belly pain and is not expecting an internal exam to be done, but is told one in fact has to be now that is the risky situation. That woman might wonder "just what is it that this doctor is up to. My problem isn't *down there*." Now *that's* a high risk situation.

I remember my secretary once asking me if I was jealous of the fact that my wife, also a physician, spends her days with naked men. Well, nearly naked anyhow (they *are* wearing underwear). I had never even thought about it before. As far as I knew the only naked man she had been around was me.

I was quite taken aback by her question. And surprised that it had never occurred to me. So I did what people typically do when asked a question they are ill prepared for and don't know the answer to. I responded immediately and with conviction. "Of course not," I said. Reflecting afterward I realized that my answer was, in fact, true.

So what is it then that makes the notion of sexual intimacy so foreign to a situation where it should be inherent? I am routinely with nearly naked women, just the two of us, behind closed doors yet the idea of this being a sexually intimate scenario seems preposterous, even bizarre. One day the answer literally walked in the door.

An exceptionally attractive woman was in the office having come for evaluation of abdominal pain. After obtaining her history I asked her to change into a gown and I left the room. A few minutes later, I knocked on the door and went in. She was sitting on the examining table, faded blue examining gown tied around her, paper drape covering her lap and legs. I examined her eyes. Corneas okay. Thyroid felt fine. A few moles on her back. Seemed benign. No breast lumps. Bit of a heart murmur. Abdomen looked okay. No liver enlargement. Bit of a rash on her legs — probably from shaving. Feet alright. Reflexes a bit down. I scrawled notes as I went. Having finished the exam I asked her to get dressed, left the room and waited a few minutes.

Going back into the room I sat down on a chair opposite hers and again realized that indeed she was an attractive woman. I was now again looking at *her*; not a varied collection of body parts in various degrees of health all playing peek-a-boo as they would briefly take turns poking out from windows created by manipulating the cloth gown and paper drape.

Context. It's all about context. (And a healthy dose of intellectualization doesn't hurt either).

Another thing: Most people look better with their clothes on than they do with them off. Been in a locker room recently? No intellectualization necessary.

The extent to which the context of an examination impacts on the perception of there being sexual overtones hit home a few years ago when a nurse working in the local emergency department was referred to me. As I wanted to accommodate her schedule I arranged to see her in the emerg during her next shift. I had her register and asked her to go into an examining room. To my surprise this was greeted with catcalls, hoots, and whistles from the rest of the nurses. She was going to be *undressed* with Doctor Blumer in the room. Now both she and I knew that her colleagues were just kibitzing; simply some gentle teasing going on. But it made us both feel uncomfortable. Had it been the private confines of my office there would have been no such discomfort. Context. A key.

Yet for all of that, there are indeed those doctors who, like certain well-known politicians, manage to get caught unzipped. There are two very simple reasons for this. Reason number one: the physician. Reason number two: the patient.

The Physician: A number of factors have been identified that increase a doctor's risk for sexual involvement. These were summarized in the Canadian Medical Association Journal (November 1, 1995; Drs. Golden and Brennan) and though some are self-evident, some are surprising:

i)   being a male physician
ii)   having female patients
iii)   being considerably older than one's patients
iv)   having a high level of educational and professional achievement
v)   using nonsexual touch more with patients of the opposite sex than with patients of the same sex
vi)   having previously been involved sexually with a teacher or supervisor
vii)   experiencing a life crisis
viii) engaging in substance abuse
ix)   denying the negative effects of such involvement for the patient
x)   previous sexual involvement with another patient [said to be the most important risk factor]

The Patient: Although you might think that certain traits such as manipulative behaviour, a personality disorder, alcoholism, and so forth would be more common among patients that get sexually involved with their doctors, Golden and Brennan's review of the medical literature in fact found that no specific trait "has been found to consistently increase the risk of involvement." I find that very disappointing. Why? Because it means that there is no ready excuse that the culprit physician can use to blame it all on the patient. Which in turn means that physicians, like everybody else, have to take responsibility for their own actions. No cop out available here.

The same study also gave some advice to physicians to follow "before erotic feelings arise." These features of course do not apply to every circumstance, but as a general rule of thumb doctors are advised to:

i)   never have sexual contact with patients (touching with the goal of sexual pleasure for oneself or the patient)
ii)   never date or flirt with patients
iii)   avoid socializing with patients
iv)   avoid nonclinical touching of patients
v)   never discuss one's personal sexual feelings and experiences with patients
vi)   avoid dressing in a sexually provocative manner at work

vii) when possible have support staff or the patient's relatives in the close vicinity when seeing a patient, and always when examining a patient's genitalia

For most doctors this whole business seems so preposterous that reading such a list would likely draw howls of derision or of laughter. In keeping with the subject matter, I can honestly say that the likelihood of my sharing my sexual feelings with a patient is about the same as my having spontaneous reversal of my circumcision. But, there are more than a few doctors who do get sexually involved (some studies — and I find this very hard to believe — quote figures of over 5 percent of physicians) and I think those of us who don't just can't fathom how it happens. Interestingly, one day I mentioned in casual conversation with a colleague that I found it incomprehensible that doctors could get sexually involved with patients. "Oh, I can see how it happens," was his surprising reply. A few months later his licence was lifted. I guess he truly could see how it happens.

Are there those physicians who are "normal," and simply "want to" have sex with a willing patient? Indeed there are. And it is indeed allowed. As long as the physician-patient relationship has ended. There was one case not too long ago wherein a physician and his patient decided to terminate their professional relationship and, one day later, began a social and sexual one. The physician's governing organization heard of the case and referred it to their discipline committee. They concluded that although they did not approve of or feel comfortable with what had transpired, they could find no transgression that had been technically committed. Where is Solomon when you need him?

When people seek medical attention for a headache their main concern tends to be that the headache might represent something sinister such as a brain tumour or a brain aneurism.

Brain aneurisms are well known to:

1. cause persisting, nagging headaches
2. lead to migraine attacks
3. cause blurred vision
4. cause nothing till they burst

Answer: 4. People tend to be very surprised when I tell them that a brain aneurism virtually never causes headache (or for that matter any other symptoms) until it ruptures. And when one does rupture, the headache tends to be horrible. A sudden, bursting, unbearable pain often accompanied by loss of consciousness.

Although I have looked after many sub-arachnoid hemorrhages (the medical term for a ruptured aneurism) there is one that was far and away the most harrowing.

It was my very first day on call as a "staff man" and I got called to a "code blue" (blue as in cyanosis, hence this term for a cardiac arrest) in the emergency room. A middle-aged woman was lying comatose. Her pulse was slow. Her breathing was laboured. I called for an intubation kit so that I could pass a tube into her airway. I asked for adrenaline to speed her heart up. *Come on, come on, what the hell was taking so long.* "Let's get moving!" I finally shouted to the nurses. They were usually tremendously efficient, but seemed now to be in chaos. They were rushing around, but seemed disorganized and ineffectual. Then I noticed their tears. I looked back down at the woman on the stretcher and noticed her white dress with a name tag on it. And then it dawned on me. She was one of them. Five minutes before, she had been working a shift as a nurse in that same emergency department. And now she was dying there. Horrible.

There are a number of rare causes of headache, but certainly one of the most intriguing has to be an orgasmic headache wherein immediately after orgasm a sudden severe headache occurs. Sort of puts a damper on things, I would imagine.

If you are in advanced middle age (let's say, over sixty years old) and have a persisting headache over one temple you may find your doctor asking some seemingly irrelevant questions. For example, do you get stiffness of your hands when you awaken? Do your joints hurt you? Any aching in your thighs or arms? Any fevers or weight loss?

What disease would be suggested by symptoms such as these?

1. rheumatoid arthritis
2. depression
3. cancer
4. temporal arteritis

Answer: 4. A steady pain over one temple, particularly in the setting of systemic symptoms like those noted above, is typical of temporal arteritis. This is a condition wherein the temporal artery (which overlies the temple) is inflamed.

What causes temporal arteritis?

1. A virus
2. A bacteria

3. An immune defect
4. How the hell should I know?

Answer: 4. Look, do yourself and your doctor a favour. Don't ask a doctor what causes a disease. Go ahead and ask how to diagnose something. Or treat it. But please don't embarrass doctors by asking us to explain why a disease occurs. Typically we will either obfuscate or fabricate or, if we are being truthful and straightforward (we tend to do better with truthfulness than straightforwardness), we will simply admit that we don't know. Period.

Temporal arteritis is serious not so much for the presence of inflammation in a fairly minor artery, but moreover because when one artery is inflamed often so are others. And if the artery that supplies blood to the retina is inflamed it can thrombose (clot) and result in immediate and permanent blindness. Fortunately, there is treatment to prevent this from happening. Unfortunately, this is in the form of prednisone, a type of steroid, which if given long term can sometimes have side effects which compete with the underlying illness in a battle to determine which is worse — the disease or the treatment. More about prednisone later.

Chapter Four

WEIGHT LOSS, RARITY, AND BEING A STAR

Few things concern me as much as when a patient has had unexplained weight loss. Sure, a pound or two is not a big deal but if someone has noticed unexplained loss of ten or twenty pounds that triggers the alarm bells. It is often remarkably difficult to determine how much weight someone might have lost. Many people don't have scales or, if they do, their scales are often grossly inaccurate.

Not only does unexplained weight loss concern me, it also fascinates me. It is a mystery just begging to be unraveled.

Paul was a thirty-five-year-old homosexual living in Toronto who had a one-year history of malaise and thirty-pound weight loss; a considerable sum considering his weight had started out at only 155 pounds.

Based on this information, which diagnosis would be most likely?

1. AIDS
2. cancer
3. impaired nutrient absorption by the bowel ("malabsorption")
4. depression

Answer: 1. Many things can lead to weight loss. However in a young, urban, male homosexual, AIDS would certainly be the prime consideration.

Realizing that Paul might have AIDS necessitated an exploration of possible risk factors. Of course, being gay was an important point, but more specific features had to be addressed. Had he had multiple partners? Did he have anal intercourse? If so, was he the passive partner? Did he have oral sex or anal-oral sex? Asking these sorts of questions can be difficult. Certainly doctors who routinely see patients with possible AIDS quickly become quite nonchalant about this sort of thing, but physicians who only rarely encounter such problems often have quite a hard time with this. So what happens is one of three things: either they are good actors and can hide their discomfort; they are not such good actors and the patient quickly senses it and becomes equally uncomfortable; or, most commonly, the patient does not get asked these salient questions, instead just getting handed a requisition to go for an HIV test.

Although AIDS was a main consideration, other possibilities still had to be considered.

If Paul had a tremor, a fast heart beat, bulging eyes, and neck swelling the diagnosis would likely be:

1. congestive heart failure (CHF)
2. tuberculosis
3. hyerthyroidism (an over-active thyroid gland)
4. cancer

Answer: 3. These are typical findings of hyperthyroidism. In Paul's case these findings were absent.

With little else to go on, AIDS remained the working diagnosis and unfortunately, but not surprisingly, Paul's HIV antibody study came back positive.

Sheila was forty years of age. She had been feeling unwell for some time now. Years, in fact. Sheila was convinced that there was something very wrong — so convinced that over the past five years she had spent what seemed like half her waking hours visiting doctors. She had been studied up and down, inside and out, but nothing significant had ever been found. Recently, however, she had developed ten pound weight-loss and thus, her family doctor thought it time to get another consultant to see her.

When she came to see me I was not offering a second opinion; more likely a tenth. Now, being the umpteenth opinion in a case does have its advantages. If I found nothing of note, well, I would have lots of company. And if I found something of consequence I would be a star.

Doctors aren't often stars. Most of the time we are more like glorified (or sometimes vilified) technologists. We learn a craft and we employ it with varying levels of expertise. Treating high blood pressure or diabetes or removing appendices and gallbladders is not quite the same as piloting the space shuttle. Even those in the medical community doing so-called glamour work such as coronary by-pass or neurosurgery realize that much of what they do is surprisingly mundane. Therefore, it should come as no surprise that when in the midst of our daily routine we happen to come upon and diagnose a RARE disease we get excited. With some sheepishness I will even admit that finding a rare disease is exciting even if we can't treat it. And with even greater sheepishness I will further admit that finding a rare disease is fascinating even if the patient may die from it.

It's hard to explain this truth and I feel guilty about it, but that's the way it is. Lest my family practice colleagues take exception to these comments let me acknowledge that most family doctors do not feel quite the same way that consultants do. They may have known a patient and the family for years whereas a specialist may have met the patient just once or twice and thus the patient is, truth be told, more likely to be viewed as an "interesting case." May you never have the misfortune to become an interesting case (sort of the medical equivalent to the ancient Chinese curse; "may you live in interesting times").

As I mentioned earlier, Sheila had felt unwell for years, but had only recently developed some weight loss. As we spoke, she also mentioned that she had experienced palpitations (a perception of a particularly forceful and often rapid heart beat). And she had a headache a fair bit of the time. Nothing very remarkable so far.

When I examined her there was little to find except that her blood pressure was up. Not in the stratosphere but enough to make a note of it.

After finishing the examination, I told Sheila that, regrettably, I did not think that I had anything new to add to her case. But, just as she was about to leave, a thought struck me. Here was a lady who had been unwell for some time now, had recently lost some weight and complained of headaches and palpitations. Hmm.

Doctors are taught to think of horses, not zebras, when hoofbeats are heard. But could this indeed be a zebra? I asked Sheila to wait for a moment. I filled out a lab requisition and handed it to her. "Sheila, this may end up being a waste of your time, but I'd like you to give a urine sample to the lab and come back to see me in a month."

The constellation of high blood pressure, weight loss, headache, and palpitations can be caused by which of the following?

1. high taxes
2. the nightly news
3. a rare disease which Sheila is going to turn out to have
4. all of the above

Answer: 4. No surprise here.

Three weeks later a striped animal arrived on my doorstep. I felt like shouting Eureka! I had discovered that Sheila had too much adrenaline in her body. For Sheila, this was like drinking five cups of coffee an hour. Every hour. Her adrenaline level in fact was ten times higher than normal.

The rare disease that Sheila had was:

1. a pheochromoctyoma
2. Bell's Palsy
3. an insulinoma
4. anencephaly

Answer: 1. This is a generally benign tumour of an adrenal gland. Most of the time, if someone is found to have a pheochromocytoma, it has come to light because a patient is being investigated for "refractory hypertension" (that is; high blood pressure which is especially difficult to get under control).

After Sheila's tumour was removed she felt marvelous. The first time in five years. And you know what? I felt marvelous too. Statistically speaking, that was likely the last case of pheochromocytoma I'll ever see. At least knowingly. As my friend says, "just because you have never diagnosed a case of something doesn't mean you haven't seen a case of it." I think about that truism quite often. It keeps me humble. But not on that occasion.

When I see a man for evaluation of weight loss and it is not clear if he has lost a minimal or a great deal of weight, I look at his belt. In cases of significant weight loss, there will invariably be a positive notch sign. That is, one sees the mark on the belt from where it used to be done up and beside that one sees a new mark where the belt is now being done up. In especially worrisome cases a double or triple notch sign may be evident. The worst case I ever saw was one where the patient had drilled holes in his belt: he had run out of notches.

AIDS and pheochromocytoma clearly do not account for the majority of cases of weight loss that come through a doctor's office.

Which of the following is most likely to cause weight loss?

1. high blood pressure
2. gallstones
3. depression
4. atherosclerosis ("hardening of the arteries")

Answer: 3. Depression is a frequent cause of weight loss.

Many people with depression don't recognize that they are depressed even though it might be obvious to those around them. And probably because of this lack of self-insight and owing also to the still-existent stigma surrounding having depression, many patients suffering from weight loss on this basis are exceptionally reluctant to accept this possibility. I used to try to explain to them the reasons why I had concluded they were depressed, but as I mentioned in an earlier chapter, I found that most such patients were clearly very sceptical. The more I would try to explain, the more aggravated they became. It took a while, but I am indeed trainable and did eventually learn a better approach. To wit: "Mrs. Watson, I understand that you don't feel that you are depressed. And that you 'have no reason to be depressed.' But we've checked out everything else and found nothing. So why don't I send you to a psychiatrist to get their opinion. Maybe they'll tell you that I'm completely wrong. So what have you lost? An hour of your time. On the other hand, maybe they'll find something is there. Something they can help you with that I can't. Look, it could be the best use of an hour you've ever spent. Okay? Great, I'll arrange the appointment for you." *Works every time.*

Chapter Five

ABDOMINAL PAIN, CHRONIC PAIN, AND WHY
DRACULA NEEDED A DERMATOLOGIST

When someone gets belly ("abdominal") pain, most of the time it is a crampy, fleeting sort of pain readily self-diagnosed as being "cramps" and cured with the next visit to the bathroom. In other words, everybody gets occasional abdominal pain. As such, those individuals who seek medical attention for abdominal pain are generally those who have more persisting or recurring pain.

Like most other symptoms, the key to establishing a diagnosis is:

1. what you tell your doctor
2. what your doctor finds when examining you
3. what an x-ray shows
4. what is found on a blood or urine test

Answer: 1. If real estate is "location, location, location" then certainly medicine is "history, history, history." Not history in the sense of studying the ailments of ancient Greece, but rather the history of the individual's complaint. Everything else is secondary in importance. Give a vague, meandering history to a doctor who can't sort out wheat from chaff and it is guaranteed you will end up going through a heck of a lot of unnecessary investigations, not to mention wasted time and expense, before the correct diagnosis is discovered. It's like bringing your car in for repairs. Telling the mechanic that the car is pulling to the right is far more likely to lead to the diagnosis of a wheel malalignment, quick repairs, and a smaller bill than if you just say "my car's not working properly."

Belly pain that has been present for years is probably due to:

1. something that won't kill you
2. something that will kill you

Answer: 1. The longer a pain has been present, the less likely it is to be due to anything life-threatening or sinister. With very rare exceptions (thyroid cancer being one), cancers are virtually never a slowly progressive, indolent disease taking years to be discovered.

Chronic pain is awful for the patient, but it's a pain for physicians too. With rare exceptions, physicians dislike seeing patients with chronic pain syndromes. It makes us feel frustrated, insecure, and, ahem, impotent. And that emanates from the fact that we often do not know the cause (which makes us feel stupid and we don't want to feel stupid so we figure the patient is probably just a complainer and *not really in that much pain*) and can't cure the patient (which means they keep coming back to us which means we have to hear the same complaint over and over, each time being reminded we haven't found out what's wrong or even if we have we still haven't been able to do much good for the patient). And because we get frustrated by these patients they get referred to one specialist after another, which serves two purposes: one, it gets them out of the office; and two, the patient feels that we are "doing something for them."

Patients with chronic pain are often referred to rheumatologists. Some of these patients have localized pain such as in a knee due to arthritis and such patients are generally fairly easy to treat. Commonly, however, patients will have "generalized" pain. Such patients can often be diagnosed within thirty seconds of meeting them. They walk into the examining room and the very first thing they say is "I hurt all over." With rare exception they suffer from fibromyalgia (also called "fibrositis"). "Fibrositic" patients invariably complain of pain from the top of their head to the bottom of their feet. Even lightly touching their skin makes them jump. Their tests are always normal. Over one-half of all referrals to rheumatologists are made up of such patients. They are present by the millions. They are often so incapacitated that they are on long-term disability.

Actually, fibromyalgia patients are often diagnosed while they are still in the waiting room and haven't even been seen by the doctor. So how could a physician be so prescient? With a bit of help. You see, in fact it is the rheumatologist's secretary who has quickly come to learn certain typical diagnostic clues:

Clue No. 1: fibrositic patients show up early for doctor's
          appointments
Clue No. 2: fibrositic patients are well made-up (the great majority
          being female)
Clue No. 3: fibrositic patients look remarkably healthy

So what sinister factor is responsible for causing fibromyalgia? The medical literature is replete with culprits. And of course the more theories there are, the more transparent it becomes that we really have no clue what the real cause is. With one major exception. Fibrositic patients are often depressed and/or under great stress. And cannot cope with life.

Now to change direction here, let's see how you do with the following brief scenarios.

Suddenly onsetting, severe abdominal pain may be due to:

    1. gout
    2. a heart attack
    3. a stroke
    4. all of the above

Answer: 2. If a heart attack involves the lowermost part of the heart (the "inferior wall") it can cause pain in the upper part of the abdomen. And that, not infrequently, leads to a misdiagnosis. Doctors are simply not as likely to suspect a heart attack when the patient's pain is not in the chest.

Belly pain that varies in location moment to moment is typical of:

    1. appendicitis
    2. diverticulitis
    3. irritable bowel syndrome (IBS)
    4. gallstones

Answer: 3. In this condition the bowel goes into spasms. The adjective "irritable" refers to the inherent irritability of the bowel in this disease, not the personality of the sufferer. It is notable however that many patients with IBS are indeed quite irritable. This may be owing to irritable individuals being more likely to develop a spastic bowel or perhaps because a spastic bowel and its attendant pain makes someone irritable.

Burning pain that is in the upper middle (just below the breastbone — an area called the "epigastrium") of the abdomen is often due to:

1. gallstones
2. an ulcer
3. ulcerative colitis
4. hepatitis

Answer: 2.

An episodic, aching pain that bores from the epigastrium through to the middle of the back and occurs primarily after eating is a possible symptom of:

1. gallstones
2. pancreatitis
3. bowel cancer
4. prostatitis

Answer: 1.

Pancreatic cancer has all of the following features except:

1. increased risk of phlebitis
2. a good prognosis
3. jaundice
4. abdominal pain

Answer: 2. Because pancreatic cancer is typically quite advanced before it is discovered, when it is finally found there is almost never a chance for a cure. Cancer in general is bad news. Pancreatic cancer in particular is dreadful news.

Doctors learn from books, journals, and lectures. We also learn from our mistakes....

I was an intern and was on one of my first nights on call. I was asked to see a thirty-five-year-old man with pancreatic cancer. He was in severe pain. I ordered some morphine for him. It didn't help. I increased the dose. No better. I increased the dose further. Still no effect. I went back into the room and said to him "I know that you're having terrible pain, but I can't give you any more morphine. It might make you so groggy you'll stop breathing."

"I understand," he replied calmly. (*Could I ever be that calm in those circumstances?* I asked myself. I knew the answer.)

The following morning I found out that this poor man had had a miserable night. Wretched in fact. He suffered until the next day when someone finally gave him what he needed. More morphine.

I had not realized that overdosing on morphine virtually never occurs if one is still in pain. I had also not known that people quickly develop tolerance to narcotics and can easily handle doses that would be lethal in someone not accustomed to getting them.

My lack of experience had led to that man's unnecessary suffering. I was furious with myself. And I felt terribly guilty about what had happened. But I learned from it. And however horrible the experience was for that unfortunate man and however awful I felt for my own shortcomings, I promised that it would never happen again. Now, almost twenty years later I can say that it never has. Does that give me some comfort? Yes, some. Not a lot mind you, but some.

The way that pain radiates is also crucial in determining its origin. Pain radiation refers to the direction that it travels. Where it comes from and where it goes to. Does it begin in the pit of your stomach and go straight through to your back? Or does it start in your back and travel to your front? And so on.

Pain that starts in the flank, courses its way across the belly and ends in the groin is characteristic of:

1. appendicitis
2. Crohn's Disease
3. an inguinal hernia
4. kidney stones

Answer: 4. And if you have ever had kidney stones you will never forget that pain's journey. The other thing sufferers from kidney stones invariably note is that after having agonizing pain they end up peeing out a minuscule stone. No sense of proportion there. Quite similar to a heart attack, really. A major, indeed massive heart attack in fact is caused by a tiny blood clot about the size of an uncooked piece of rice.

Most of the time the way a pain radiates is in keeping with the underlying anatomy (for example, pain in the lower right area of the belly in appendicitis) however in medicine all too often things are not so straightforward — not for the doctor or for the patient. Perhaps it is to prevent doctors from becoming too complacent that studies come out showing rather inexplicable and indeed, sometimes quite bizarre results. To wit, the study wherein balloons were inserted in patients' rectums and passed up into the colon (no, I don't know where the volunteers came from) and then inflated. This was to simulate the pain felt in a spastic bowel condition. Logically, pain would be expected to occur in that area of the abdomen overlying the site of the balloon. And that did happen. But pain was also noted to radiate high up into the chest. *High up in the chest.* Amazing.

Another key characteristic of a pain's behaviour is what exacerbates it and what relieves it. Most people know, for example, that if they have burning upper abdominal pain and it is quickly eased by taking an antacid then the pain was probably due to some acid indigestion (be it from an ulcer, hiatus hernia, or whatever).

If, after consuming some ice cream, you get abdominal pain and diarrhea you may be suffering from:

1. irritable bowel syndrome
2. an ulcer
3. stomach cancer
4. lactose intolerance

Answer: 4. The natural sugar in milk products is lactose. To digest this, the human gut is rich in an enzyme called lactase. If you lack this enzyme, after consuming milk-containing products lactose builds up in the bowel and has a toxic effect, leading to abdominal pain and diarrhea. This seems straightforward enough. And it is. Where it gets tricky, however, is when patients being investigated for diarrhea deny consuming any milk products. Playing detective will sometimes allow the discovery that they were unknowingly taking milk products in the form of cream in coffee, butter on toast, etc. On the other hand, a recent study suggested that small doses of lactose do not cause symptoms in lactose intolerant individuals. So, like much else in medicine, who really knows....

Certain positions can also influence pain. People with pancreatic cancer often find that sitting up and leaning forward is preferable to being supine. In the midst of a gallbladder attack ("biliary colic") patients often get up and pace the floor, finding it intolerable to stay still. Walking the floor doesn't actually ease the pain, but nonetheless it's what people with gallbladder attacks do. The opposite is true of the pain of acute appendicitis in which case people will prefer to lay motionless.

This, however, is easier to understand since when the appendix is inflamed, if you move around it causes the tissues overlying the appendix to rub against it — rubbing it the wrong way, so to speak.

The man upon whom the novel _Dracula_ is based was a Romanian prince named Vlad Tepes, more commonly known as Vlad the Impaler. He was disfigured and likely had recurring bouts of abdominal pain triggered by sun exposure. It is thought, therefore, that he probably had:

1. porphyria
2. desperate need of a dermatologist
3. vitiligo
4. hemophilia

Answer: 1. "2" is also acceptable. Porphyria is a rare, metabolic disease, and as noted above, causes recurring belly pain triggered by sun exposure. No surprise, therefore, that Dracula would have been a nocturnal figure.

After obtaining a history there is, of course, an examination. When doing a physical exam, there is a tendency to act like the infamous bank robber Willie Sutton and "go where the money is." That is, if someone has abdominal pain, immediately direct your attention to that area. However, to do so is unwise for it would prevent obtaining an overview of things. A _gestalt_ so to speak. For example, someone with abdominal pain due to cancer may well have a normal abdominal exam with the diagnosis therefore being delayed or possibly overlooked altogether if one does not step back and look at the whole patient. Are they pale (as they might be if anemic from a bleeding tumour), jaundiced (if they had metastases to the liver), or cachectic (as is typical of many cancers)? These key clues can be missed if one gets too focused just on the symptomatic area.

Similarly, we have to look over the entire abdomen regardless of the specific location of the pain. Hopefully the patient does not take careful observation as being simple staring. People tend to feel uncomfortable when a doctor stands at the bedside just looking.

Without even laying a hand on the abdomen some things can be apparent, such as scars ("Oh, Mrs. Jones did you have your appendix out?" "Yes, doctor, I forgot to mention it before"), distension (such as might be seen with a collection of gas or fluid), stretch marks (which can, of course, occur with pregnancy, but can also be seen with a condition of excess cortisol hormone), gross enlargement of the liver (noted in the right upper area of the abdomen), or spleen (noted in the left upper area of the abdomen). All this from just a look. Like the song says, "Just one look, that's all it takes...."

I've also discovered that the great majority of woman who have had breast reduction surgery ("reduction mammoplasty") never mention it during the interview — only when I examine them is it revealed. Forgetfulness? Embarrassment? Perhaps forgetting that which is embarrassing?

Text books routinely use the expression "using the *gloved* finger" when referring to the technique for performing a rectal examination. This is:

    1. true
    2. false
    3. I must be joking

Answer: 1. No joke. Go figure.

Chapter Six

BACK PAIN, DEATH, AND KNIGHTS IN WHITE DRESSES

"My back aches."

Debbie had just come off another twelve-hour nursing shift, the majority of it having been spent on her feet. She would often have to lift patients and, like many nurses, she had managed to "strain her back" — which really means she had stretched one or more of her back muscles beyond the point of contentedness. And that is far and away the most common form of back pain that physicians encounter. There are, however, many other forms of back pain, and these can be a lot harder to sort out.

Some people present to the doctor with back pain that is disproportionately severe to the findings on examination and x-ray testing. Such patients have often injured themselves at work and are not infrequently on long term disability. Because objective findings are few yet the patients' subjective findings are great, compassionate doctors will tell such patients: "pain is what the patient feels; your pain therefore is obviously real even if I can't find much to explain it." What those same doctors may then say in the doctors lounge is: "I saw another one of those disability cases. What a crock. If they were self-employed they'd have gone back to work ages ago." It is a coincidence that my office window has a bird's eye view of the parking lot. It is not, however, a coincidence that with surprising regularity I will observe "disabled" young patients who, having just hobbled out of my office, will then walk briskly across the parking lot and jump into their pickup truck.

It can be quite a game trying to separate out the people with "organic" back pain from those with "functional" back pain. To doctors, "organic" means "real." whereas "functional" means, to put it gently, less real. Not to say out-and-out fakery, but rather that someone's symptoms are a lot more "mental" than they are "physical." Which, of course, if you ask a doctor, does not mean that the pain is less legitimate, or less severe, or less important. Unless of course you hear doctors talking to one another, in which case that would be exactly what they mean.

One good trick (crass, eh?) to distinguish functional back pain from organic back pain is to ask the patient to stand then to bend at the waist as far forward as possible. In both functional and organic back pain the amount of flexion is invariably quite limited. Later in the exam, with the patient lying flat on their back, you ask them to sit up so that you can check their blood pressure. No big deal. Up they come with arm extended for a blood pressure reading. At least no big deal for the functional ones who are now sitting with their waist bent to exactly the same degree that they were totally unable to do moments before when they had been standing. The organic patient takes quite a bit longer to sit up as they twist and turn to minimize their pain.

Another form of back pain is localized to the "costo-vertebral angle"; that is, the region just below the lowest rib and just beside the back bone. The affected individual will often have a fever, may have sweats (in medical parlance a "sweat" is a sudden drenching sweat as opposed to being "sweaty" which is a more continual, less intense form of sweating) and often has uncontrollable shaking chills known as "rigors." Such a patient will often have burning when passing their urine ("dysuria") and the urine is frequently foul smelling.

Given such a scenario the likely diagnosis is:

1. cystitis (a bladder infection)
2. pyelonephritis (a kidney infection)
3. diverticulitis (inflammation of a diverticulum [a pocket or pouch coming off the bowel])
4. pelvic inflammatory disease (e.g. gonorrhea)

Answer: 2. The main distinguishing features separating a simple bladder infection from a more serious kidney infection are the lack of systemic complaints (fever, sweats, etc.) in the former. Also, back pain is highly unlikely to occur with an uncomplicated bladder infection.

Kidney infections are virtually always caused by bacteria. Despite popular wisdom to the contrary, a mild ache in the area overlying a kidney is not due to a "cold in the kidney" and is not brought on by "a draft." People do not get colds from being in a draft. And their kidneys do not get colds from being in a draft. And there is no such thing as a cold of the kidneys. Now lest I sound too dogmatic and perhaps somewhat condescending let me hasten to add the disclaimer that I use when talking to many of my patients about things in the world of medicine: "everything I tell you is based on the current medical literature." In other words, if a new study comes out later proving that I was totally wrong and you, in fact, were right all along, well, don't blame me. You know, maybe tomorrow we'll find out that drafts do cause colds. But for now, it is not proven and how could anyone think such a thing.

Speaking about getting things wrong reminds me of one way in which I have observed some physicians deal with errors they have made: They simply blame the patient. To wit:

Physician interviews and examines patient. Makes diagnosis. Prescribes treatment. Patient doesn't improve. Physician talks to patient again. Physician realizes overlooked key information.

"Why didn't you tell me that before?!" physician demands. Unsaid by physician: *"Oh hell, how did I miss that?"*

"Oh, I don't know. I'm sorry." Unsaid by patient: *"Come on now. I told you all that before. You just weren't paying attention. Don't blame me, you shmuck."*

Also familiar to lay and medical people alike is the frequent, at times continual aching in the back generally found in older people and due to osteoarthritis ("degenerative arthritis"). It's the price we homo sapiens pay for evolution having allowed us to walk upright. Being bipeds, our backs must bear the wear and tear inflicted upon by our weight. And that repetitive stress takes its toll by way of causing the back bone to degenerate. Such degenerative arthritis has even been found in dinosaur bones.

If I were to ask you what it would suggest if a patient came to a hospital complaining of severe "tearing" pain travelling from the upper back down to the lower back you might well reply it suggests that something is:

1. tearing
2. not tearing

Answer: 1. Now since when is anything in medicine as straightforward as it seems? Well, sometimes it is. The aorta is the body's main artery (arteries carry blood from the heart to the rest of the body; veins carry blood from the body back to the heart) and on occasion, particularly in elderly individuals, a tear may form in the aorta and then spread down the vessel. It causes an excruciating, ripping pain in the back.

It was a Saturday in January and I was stuck on call yet again. I was summoned to the emergency department to see a young woman who had come in with back pain. It sounded routine enough until I was told that Mrs. Robinson had a history of breast cancer. Now if there is anything that is guaranteed to make a doctor's light bulb turn on it is the presence of new pain in someone known to have or to have had cancer. Mrs. Robinson's pain had come on fairly recently and was progressively worsening. She had to resort to taking Tylenol with codeine to get some relief.

Some key questions are raised in this circumstance. Particularly important are those pertaining to:

1. blood pressure
2. earache
3. leg weakness
4. gout

Answer: 3. It is crucial to know if there are any associated neurological symptoms and in particular if there is any leg weakness. If there is a metastatic deposit in the vertebral column (the "back bone") it might be pressing on the spinal cord and that would be a true medical emergency. Undue delay and the patient might become paralyzed. I thought of this as I palpated Mrs. Robinson's spine.

I pressed on Mrs. Robinson's upper thoracic spine. No problem. Seventh thoracic vertebrae OK. T8 OK. T9, T10, T11, all OK. Then my stomach turned over. I felt like I was going to be sick. I was pressing on T12 but there wasn't one. Just mush. And as I pressed, Mrs. Robinson said where I was touching was sore and that her right leg had just got a numb, shooting pain. She turned her head and looked up at me.

"Is everything all right?" she asked, knowing that everything was not all right but hoping otherwise.

"Well," I began, not knowing quite how to answer, "I think there is some irritation in your back."

"What does that mean?" she asked.

I debated how I was going to answer. I think that beating around the bush is inappropriate. Patients invariably recognize evasiveness for what it is and assume the worst. Contrariwise, being overly blunt can border on the cruel and inhumane. I tried a middle ground. "I think that the back pain you are experiencing is due to some inflammation in your spine." I hoped that would suffice for the time being. It didn't.

"Doctor, just what are you saying?" she replied. I took a deep breath.

"I am concerned that your back pain may be there because of spread of your breast cancer."

A terrible and terrifying and terrified look came across her face. Then came a flood of tears. Hers. I held mine back.

I never find it easy to impart terrible news. And each time I do I keep trying to word things better than the time before hoping that I will eventually come across just the right way of saying things. But I never feel that it comes out quite right. And I'm sure that is because I want it be painless. Painless for the patient. Painless for the family. And probably painless for me. But it never is. And I guess it never could be. You know, I'm sort of glad it never is painless for me. If it were, I bet it would be time to change careers.

There is one way that doctors can try to escape from the responsibility of imparting bad news. They slough the responsibility onto somebody else's shoulders. Let's say, for example, that someone goes to see their general practitioner because of some rectal bleeding. The doctor does a rectal exam and feels a mass. He tells the patient that "there is something that seems abnormal in the rectum." The "Big C" (the ultimate euphemism for cancer) is never mentioned. The patient gets referred to an internist who does a scoping procedure on the bowel (sigmoidoscopy) and sees a big, fungating mass. He tells the patient that "there appears to be a tumour," but conveniently fails to mention that it looks overwhelmingly like a cancer. He then tells the patient that he will have to see a surgeon. The surgeon repeats the scope and does a biopsy. It comes back confirming what all the doctors had suspected all along — cancer. The surgeon is the lucky one that then gets to impart the grim news to the patient.

The previous physicians had both suspected cancer, but had not mentioned it. The justification for this is that the diagnosis was uncertain and why would you worry a patient needlessly? Except that it is a rare patient indeed that would not have already spent considerable time worrying that this "mass" was a cancer. Not raising this with the great majority of patients just feeds into their fears and reinforces the notion that cancer is a four letter word — best not to even mention it; never mind talking about it. No, the real reason many doctors don't raise the spectre of cancer until it is biopsy-proven, even when there is near certainty of its presence, is because of cowardice. To raise the issue would then require a detailed discussion of prognosis, treatment, and so forth.

And most physicians would rather hide than to have to tell a patient that they likely have a potentially fatal disease. So it's left to the last doctor on the referral chain — generally the surgeon — to deal with.

But sometimes even the surgeon chickens out. What happens is that the surgeon performs an operation, establishes a diagnosis, and relates it to the patient, but fails to then proceed on to the next logical step. That is, explaining to the patient key pieces of information that will directly affect their prognosis. Were any lymph glands involved by the tumour? Was there evidence of a tumour in the resection line (that is, at the outer edge of the removed tissue)? And also conveniently ignored are the unasked questions that patients are afraid to voice. *Am I cured? What are the chances it will come back? If it recurs, how am I likely to notice? Will I be in pain? Will I suffer? Am I going to die?* Questions unasked. Questions unanswered. The doctor may know these questions are there, but are unspoken. Easier not to deal with them at all.

When a doctor tells someone horrible news, the reaction is generally what you would expect. Tears, grief, denial, and the rest of the gamut. What I see less often is anger. Anger directed at me.

I was in the emergency department when a twenty-five-year-old man was brought in following an explosion that occurred while he was working on a hydro-electric transformer. Taking one look at him it was obvious that things were pretty grim. We tried to resuscitate him, but it was hopeless. After the "code was called" (medicalese meaning resuscitation efforts were abandoned) it was up to me to talk to his wife. The idea of telling her that her husband had just suddenly and unexpectedly died made me cringe. I asked the nurse to put the wife, a very large young woman, in a quiet room and the equally large nurse and I entered after her. I introduced myself and we all sat down.

"I'm very sorry ..." I started to say, but was interrupted.

"Don't tell me," she glared. "Don't tell me. He isn't. He's not ..."

If I told her he was dead, he was. If I kept quiet, there was still hope.

"I'm very sorry," I began again, "you're husband has died." As I said these words I wondered if it would have been gentler to have said "you're husband has passed away" or "you're husband didn't make it" or some such thing, but I kept hearing this voice in my ear from lecturers past: "be direct, don't beat around the bush, don't use euphemisms, if someone has died say so."

An instant after I said the word "died" she launched from her chair. Smack, my head flinched to the left. Smack, my head veered to the right. I was so startled it didn't even occur to me to defend myself. As the next blow was inches from my face, my knight in a white dress seized the woman's arm in mid-air and, saviour that she was, hugged her. Not a little hug, but a great big bear of a hug. And put the woman's head on her shoulder. Where she sobbed for her loss.

A bit later, after the wife had gone into her dead husband's room, I approached Lise, the nurse, and remarked on how compassionate she had been. "Compassion? Hell no. I knew if I didn't hug her she would have beat the crap out of you."

A cop who had come to investigate the death heard what had happened to me, looked at my increasingly swollen face, and to my amazement, asked me if I wanted to press charges.

"Huh?" or some equally brilliant thing, I muttered.

"Charges. Do you want to press charges?" he asked again.

"Against who?" I asked (I wasn't up to being grammatically correct).

"That lady, the one that hit you," the cop said, obviously thinking I was a dolt of the highest order.

"No, no, uhh, of course not," I managed to get out. "She has gone through a lot more than I have." I didn't feel like a hero for saying that. I felt like a shmuck for having done such a lousy job of telling this woman her husband had died.

To that unfortunate woman I surely had been the enemy. The Grim Reaper. Sometimes, though, it is the other way around and the patient is perceived as being the enemy. How so? Thought you'd never ask....

Let's say that it's ten o'clock on a Saturday evening. You've been feeling unwell all day with recurring episodes of an abdominal pain which, though not severe, are nonetheless worrying you so you decide, after some prompting from your spouse, that you should get it checked out. Living in an urban area you have a nearby teaching hospital to which you then go. The emergency department is busy, but eventually you are taken in and, around midnight, you get seen by the emergency room physician who decides that you should see the surgery resident.

Around two in the morning, the surgery resident arrives. His manner is brusk. He asks you a few pointed questions and pokes your belly. He then tells you it's "nothing" and, without a good-bye, he turns on his heels and walks away.

"What a rude bastard," you think to yourself.

Getting home, you climb into bed and, your pain having settled, you drift off to sleep.

Morning comes and your friend, who happens to be a physician, is over for brunch.

"You know Jeff, I was in the emerg last night because of some belly pain. Saw this young guy, probably just out of medical school. What a prick! Spent two seconds with me, told me there was nothing wrong and left the room. I didn't know whether he was coming back, going to order tests or what. I lay there like a putz until a nurse came by and told me I could go home. I feel okay now, but I can tell you right now there's no way in hell I'm ever going back to that hospital."

Jeff, a physician for the past fifteen years, listens to your diatribe and responds. "That's not really a surprise you know. To that doctor you were the enemy."

"The enemy. How the hell was I the enemy? I was there to get help. Not to cause problems."

"Doesn't matter. That guy who saw you had likely been working since seven in the morning. If he was lucky he might have had an hour or two of sleep before they woke him up to come see you. And he probably knew he wouldn't get any more sleep because the emerg was busy and they would probably have more patients for him. And in a few hours he likely had to start his ward rounds."

"So what, he's getting paid for it. It's his job. Look, I think there's no excuse for that sort of behaviour."

"I really don't want to sound like an apologist for this guy. Maybe he was an obnoxious putz, pure and simple. But I just want you to realize that he was likely exhausted, had been run off his feet all day and, you know, he doesn't get paid extra to see you. A resident's salary isn't great to start with. And they get paid the same if they work one hour or twenty-four hours in a day. So what incentive is there? Why should he be happy to be called back to the emerg at two in the morning? He would rather have been at home asleep."

"Jeff, you *do* sound like an apologist. Why do you doctors always rush to defend each other? This guy was rude. He was obnoxious. And I don't think there's any excuse for it."

"You're right. He does sound rude and obnoxious. And I agree it's not right. But I'm not trying to justify it, just to explain it."

"Okay, okay. I see what you're saying. Want some more coffee?"

"Sure."

"Oh Jeff, one other thing."

"Uhuh?"

"Were you like that guy when you were a resident?"

"Me? Of course not. I was always charming."

"Bull."

"Yup. Bull."

Chapter Seven

FEVER, GLAMOUR, AND FEARING THE LIGHTS

I love seeing patients with fever. But not just any fever. It has to be at least 100.5 °F. And it has to have been present for at least a week. That will eliminate the great majority of self-limited viral illnesses. So many symptoms are so nebulous that it can be a real treat to have something concrete to evaluate; something which must be "organic." Especially if you are an internist.

I am an internist. That is not the same as an intern. Believe me. An intern is a newly graduated physician who is completing basic post-graduate training before either going into a general practice or taking further training to become a specialist. An internist is an individual who has completed an internship and has then gone on to complete anywhere from three to five additional years of specialty training.

The concept of an internist is elusive. I have tried to define what I do in many different ways, but it never seems to come across as clearly as I would like. Physician associations in Canada and the United States have had similar difficulties. I *can* say that an internist is a physician who, on a referral basis, assesses patients with regard to a *medical* problem usually affecting one of the major internal organs. We do not do surgery. We do not do dermatology. Nor psychiatry, otorhinolaryngology (diseases of the ear, nose, and throat), or gynecology. We do see people with heart problems such as angina or heart failure, people with lung problems such as asthma or bronchitis, people with bowel troubles such as constipation or diarrhea. Straightforward? If so, then I am being too cut and dry about it. Because ...

We actually often *do* see people with skin rashes because they can be associated with internal diseases (such as a facial rash in lupus). And we *do* perform certain quasi-surgical procedures such as endoscopy (peering into one of a variety of orifices with fiberoptic scopes) and organ biopsies. And to make it especially confusing, in the United States internists often *do* gynecology and often *do* primary care. I have not yet come up with a satisfactory definition as to exactly what it is I do. My father still calls me regularly to find out.

Oh, and by the way, if ever you have the (mis?)fortune to see an internist please, please don't ask if he/she is an intern. It's highly insulting. And we're a very defensive lot.

That aside aside, let us return to our discussion of fever.

One key point to establish is the character of the fever. How long has it been there? How high does it go? Does it spike up and down several times per day or is it a low grade, fairly constant elevation? Does it ever go away for a day or more? And so on.

Patricia Reynoldson, a fifty-five-year-old woman, comes into the hospital with appendicitis. She is taken to the operating room and has what appears to be uneventful surgery. Three days later she develops a fever of 101 °F. The nurse becomes concerned about Mrs. Reynoldson and calls the surgeon.

En route to the ward, which of the following possible explanations for the patient's fever does the surgeon consider?

1. phlebitis
2. an abscess in the abdomen
3. pneumonia
4. all of the above
5. none of the above

Answer: 4.

The surgeon arrives on the ward and examines Mrs. Reynoldson. Although the patient's lungs sound fine, the doctor orders a chest x-ray anyhow.

She did this because:

1. her friend is a financially strapped radiologist
2. she is too lazy to thoroughly examine the patient's lungs
3. she knows that a normal lung exam does not exclude pneumonia
4. she wants to make sure there is not an abscess under the diaphragm

Answer: 3. (Not to be too cynical, but I wouldn't completely exclude 2 [half marks if you chose this number]. Number 1 is reputed not to exist.)

Mrs. Reynoldson's chest x-ray comes back normal. The surgeon therefore decides that pneumonia is not present and goes back to reassess the patient. On doing so she finds that the patient's abdomen is soft and non-tender.

This is reassuring because it:

1. makes it unlikely that there is an abscess in the abdomen
2. makes it less likely that the surgeon's malpractice premiums are going to rise
3. means it is not a surgical problem (which translates into "nurse, please get the internist on call to see the patient")
4. all of the above

Answer: 4. No surprise here.

The esteemed (ahem) internist arrives on the scene. He reviews the chart (definitely not a surgeon), gets more detailed information on the patient's progress from the nurse (ditto), talks to the patient and then examines her top to bottom (ditto again). Needless to say, internists have a well-founded reputation for obsessive behaviour. He notes that she is now three days post-operative, has a low-grade fever, and that her left calf is a bit sore and swollen.

He decides that the most likely cause of Mrs. Reynoldson's fever is:

1. a torn calf muscle
2. gout
3. phlebitis
4. a reaction to a drug

Answer: 3.

This is a classical story for phlebitis (which, you may recall, is defined as a blood clot in a vein). There are a number of risk factors including recent surgery, obesity, smoking, use of the birth control pill, pregnancy, and a family history of phlebitis.

Given that we are dealing with a classical story for phlebitis, no further investigations are necessary. This is:

1. true
2. false

Answer: 2. false.

With a textbook, classical, convincing, straightforward, obvious, and unequivocal presentation for phlebitis, the likelihood that a patient in fact actually has the condition is about:

1. 100%
2. 90%
3. 80%
4. 50%

Answer: 4. When you are completely certain that a patient has phlebitis you should think again. Indeed, you may as well flip a coin.

The gold-standard test to decide if someone has phlebitis is:

1. impedence plethysmography (try dropping that term at a party)
2. doppler ultrasonography
3. venography

Answer: 3. A venogram entails placing a needle into the foot and injecting dye into the veins. It is without a doubt the most accurate test for evaluating possible phlebitis however it does have some risk to it (how about this for example; a venogram to detect phlebitis can actually cause phlebitis!) and thus other studies like those listed above are often done in its place.

Mrs. Reynoldson has a venogram and phlebitis is confirmed. The test result therefore is considered:

1. positive
2. negative

Answer: 1. Half marks for choice 2. It's a matter of perspective and semantics, isn't it? A "positive" result is certainly "negative" for the patient, is it not?

As most of the lay world knows, physicians are a cohesive, unified group. As most physicians know, unity amongst doctors lasts until the conversation turns from how much we dislike the Ministry of Health (*any* Ministry of Health) to any other subject, including the weather.

If you will now please imagine an introductory drum roll, I will then follow that with a capsule summary of doctors' personality traits as defined by their specialty.

Internists (be they general internists or subspecialists thereof such as cardiologists, lung specialists, and so on) think surgeons are technicians, not thinkers. Internists think surgeons are scalpel happy. Internists think surgeons are rude, arrogant, and generally obnoxious. Internists get mad at the undue attention that the press lavishes on surgeons. Internists get mad at the fact that surgery is considered "sexy." Internists secretly long to be surgeons.

Surgeons think that internists spend so much time "thinking," that they never make up their minds about anything, and that they never actually "do" anything. Surgeons think they are superior to internists, and everyone else for that matter. Surgeons love attention and glory. Surgeons know they are "sexy." Surgeons secretly long to be movie stars.

Internists and surgeons do agree on one key point. They're both glad they're not psychiatrists.

Psychiatrists think they are the only ones that really, truly understand the inner workings of their patients. Psychiatrists think the psyche and the body are inseparable. Psychiatrists know that internists also say that the psyche and the body are inseparable, but don't really mean it. Psychiatrists hate the fact that they are near the bottom of the medical pay scale. Psychiatrists would make lousy surgeons. Surgeons would make even worse psychiatrists. Psychiatrists secretly long to be Sigmund Freud, but know that would mean being well over one hundred years old and besides he never did understand women and leather couches are so expensive anyhow and who wants to move to Austria and gee, well, I guess it's better not to be him after all, when you really think about it.

Family doctors think they are the only ones that really, truly understand the inner workings of their patients. Family doctors hate that they are at the bottom of the pay scale. Family doctors are jealous of the fact that specialists are considered sexier than they. Family doctors "don't get no respect." Family doctors can "bounce" their "chronic complainers" only so far and for so long before they come back. Family doctors care more about their patients than any specialists could. Family doctors are a God-send to the rest of doctors. Family doctors secretly long to be specialists; excepting that specialists are a bunch of pedantic, over-paid, long-winded shmucks.

All doctors wish that they were in charge — of everything. All doctors think they know more than anyone else — about anything. All doctors wish that they had the neat monitors in the sick bay of the U.S.S. *Enterprise*. All doctors are smart. Many doctors are not clever. All doctors wish they were more knowledgeable, more respected, better paid, less over-worked, and less stressed. All doctors should have a periodic reality check. All doctors say that they don't want to play God. All doctors wish that they *were* God.

Now that I have undoubtedly raised the temperature of sufficient numbers of my colleagues to cause a surge in global warming, let us return to our discussion about fever.

One of the most recognizable fever patterns is the daily "spiking" of a high temperature as is characteristic of an abscess. Quite differently, Hodgkin's Disease can cause fevers lasting a few days alternating with several day periods free of fever. No fever pattern, however, can be considered pathognomonic (being so characteristic of a particular disease so as to clinch the diagnosis based solely on the one feature).

As with other symptoms, we have to look at the company fever keeps. It is important to determine if there are shaking chills ("rigors") and sweats. Rigors and sweats are typically seen in bacterial infections. Sweats without rigors can be seen with a variety of illnesses including lymph gland tumours or leukemias (cancerous proliferation of the white blood cells).

If you report to your doctor that you are having weight loss, persisting fevers and night sweats and he or she doesn't quickly get interested, you should:

1. call an undertaker (the doctor must be dead)
2. change doctors

Answer: 1 and 2 are both right.

You are an emergency room physician. A nurse hands you the chart on a patient who has come to the hospital with a three-hour history of fever.

Before you get any additional information you already realize that:

1. this patient is probably very sick
2. you're about to make an easy thirty bucks
3. pneumonia is a main consideration
4. it is probably "the flu"

Answer: 1. Very, very few people, even the most neurotic of individuals, are likely to come to hospital after having had a fever for only a few hours. To have done so, this patient is probably profoundly ill.

You go into the patient's cubicle (and for those of you familiar with emergency departments you will immediately recognize the accuracy of that term) to assess him. But as you enter you can barely see him because the lights are off.

With not a word spoken and not a hand laid on the patient you already know that this man probably has:

1. a migraine headache
2. the flu
3. a room with a broken lightbulb
4. meningitis

Answer: 4. Sudden development of profound illness with fever and photophobia (technically defined as a "fear of lights," but in practice not a fear but simply a preference to avoid lights) is awfully suspicious for meningitis. And not just any meningitis, but the most severe kind: bacterial.

Some additional scenarios:

A fifty-year-old man presents with a fever, cough, greenish/yellow sputum, and pain on breathing ("pleurisy"). He probably has:

1. bronchitis
2. pneumonia
3. emphysema
4. pericaridits

Answer: 2.

A thirty-five-year-old woman has fever, right-sided back pain, burning discomfort when passing urine ("dysuria") and her urine smells bad. She probably has:

1. pyelonephritis (kidney infection)
2. cystitis (bladder infection)
3. gonorrhea
4. a ruptured ovarian cyst

Answer: 1. If you got this wrong then you weren't paying attention during the previous chapter. If so, then don't worry, it is reassuring that it is not only medical students that daydream while reading medical books.

A twenty-five-year-old man just returned from Mexico is feverish and is passing a dozen loose stools per day. The likely diagnosis is:

1. alcohol over-indulgence
2. typhoid fever
3. diverticulitis
4. traveller's diarrhea

Answer: 4. This is a bowel infection and can be due to quite a variety of different organisms including bacteria such as salmonella and campylobacter.

Some causes of fever are not nearly so straightforward. Indeed, some of the most challenging cases of my career have been patients suffering from febrile illnesses. One of these patients was Kim, an eighteen-year-old woman who presented with a month-long history of fever, sweats, twenty-pound weight loss, generalized weakness, and malaise. She was sure she had some sinister disease. I must admit I shared her concern.

I investigated her top to bottom. Inside and out. Nothing. Sometimes nothing is good, but not when the patient is very ill.

I checked Kim for bacterial infections. None. For AIDS. Not there. For Hodgkin's Disease. No. There was no evidence of a factitious fever (there are indeed those individuals who will hold a thermometer under hot water in order to simulate a fever). Day after day went by without a diagnosis. She looked increasingly unwell. Her weight kept falling. Her complexion sallowed and she became increasingly anemic.

I kept reminding myself of the wisdom (there wasn't much of it but some pearls did emerge) imparted to us in medical school. The first step in assessing a patient is to do a history and physical. And if things do not become clear thereafter, do it again. And again. I did as I had been taught. Still nothing.

I spoke to colleagues, read textbooks and reviewed journal articles, but all to no avail. I felt increasingly discouraged. *Why couldn't I figure out her problem? What kind of doctor was I anyhow?* Fragile ego rearing its head.

My father, in reference to my abilities as a physician, once asked me if I ever felt "cocky."

"No," I answered, and I was thinking about Kim as I replied. Indeed, how can any physician ever feel so overwhelmingly confident as to be "cocky." Such an individual would surely be dangerous. Medicine is as much art as science. And there are few absolutes in science, and fewer still in the arts. That leaves no room for cockiness. When patients rave to me about the "very confident" doctor they just saw I always hope that the physician's confidence is equalled by similarly strong inquisitiveness and at least a small but significant measure of self-doubt.

Kim had now been ill for what seemed like an eternity. Yet she had defied diagnosis. Daily, I would sit down and retake her history, re-examine her, and pour over her chart reviewing all the laboratory data, x-ray results, nuclear scans, and so forth, hoping some faint glimmer of light would emerge.

And then, hallelujah, one day it did. In the unlikely form of a skin rash.

A skin rash may not sound like a very exciting finding given all the other symptoms that she had been having, but I can tell you with great conviction that after wracking your brains out and getting nowhere, any new clue, and especially something concrete and objective like a skin rash, is heaven-sent.

It is rare that an urgent dermatology consultation is required but that was indeed just what the doctor (ahem) ordered.

A skin biopsy was obtained and lo and behold the report came back showing "a neutrophilic infiltrate of the endothelium with some necrosis and small thrombus material." That medicalese gobbledygook told me that the patient was suffering from:

1. vasculits
2. retinitis pigmentosa
3. candidiasis
4. environmental allergy syndrome

Answer: 1. Vasculitis means inflammation of the blood vessels. The biopsy report showed a "neutrophilic" (neutrophils are a type of white blood cell) infiltrate of the "endothelium" (the inner lining of blood vessels) with some "necrosis" (destroyed tissue) and small "thrombus" (blood clot) material. In other words, the biopsy showed typical changes of inflammation of a blood vessel.

And to treat inflammation, what better drug than an anti-inflammatory agent? In this case a powerful one known as prednisone. Within twenty-four hours Kim's fever had resolved, her appetite had improved, and she was well on the road to recovery. And I started to sleep better. I was very proud of myself. And I felt a bit cocky. Oops.

Chapter Eight

JOINT PAIN, LOVE, AND DRUG COMPANY REPS

J oint pains have been around for as long as there have been joints. And that's a long time. The most common form of joint pain is due to degenerative arthritis, also known as osteoarthritis or by the somewhat more apt term *wear and tear* arthritis. We all get it as we age. Often the small joints in our fingers will become somewhat misshapen and it may be difficult to do activities such as writing, hammering, etc. The back, hips, and knees are also frequently affected.

Like most things in medicine, the cause of osteoarthritis is not clear-cut. To wit: we call it wear and tear arthritis because we assume that repetitive stress on a joint is the culprit. That helps us to understand why, for instance, a football player might get it in his knees. But surely the strain on the knees in a 250-pound athlete cannot be compared with the stress on a finger joint in an eighty-year-old knitter. But the same disease process appears in both.

One of the most difficult things to explain to patients is the difference between osteoarthritis and rheumatoid arthritis. They differ in that rheumatoid arthritis:

1. typically begins in younger people

2. does not have as much inflammation
3. is more likely to involve the back
4. is caused by damp weather

Answer: 1.

Osteoarthritis can affect virtually any joint in the body whereas rheumatoid arthritis affects primarily the small joints of the hands and feet and to a lesser extent larger joints such as the knees, elbows, and ankles. They both can lead to deformity but that related to rheumatoid arthritis tends to be more severe. Osteoarthritis, given our living long enough, will affect us all whereas rheumatoid arthritis affects only a small percentage of the population.

I used to explain to patients that one of the main differences between osteoarthrits and rheumatoid arthritis was that pain due to the former was owing to the mechanical grinding of one bone on the other whereas pain due to the latter was related to inflammation within the joint.

That explanation worked for a while, but like all simple explanations it was doomed to failure. The reason? Patients with osteoarthritis could not understand why, having just heard that they do not suffer from an inflammatory process, they were then put on an anti-inflammatory medication. These are known as NSAIDs (Non-Steroidal Anti-Inflammatory Drugs), of which there are many including such well-known ones as Motrin (Ibuprofen) or Indocid (Indomethacin).

Why an anti-inflammatory drug for a non-inflammatory condition? Good question. I wish there was an equally good answer. Actually, part of the rationale is that NSAID drugs can act as analgesics regardless of the disease they are being used to treat. More importantly, even so-called non-inflammatory arthritis often does have some degree of inflammation and thus there is the potential for response to this form of therapy. There tends not to be a great response, but there can be some.

Which of the following side effects are anti-inflammatory drugs well known to cause?

a) impotence
b) stomach ulcers
c) epilepsy
d) kidney failure

Choose either: 1. a) and c)
2. b) and d)

3. none of the above (out of principal because multiple-multiple choice questions remind you of the ridiculous, nightmarish questions you thought were gone forever once you finished school and you have vowed to never answer another one for the rest of your life and you believe in sticking by your convictions because you are a very principled individual)

Answer: 2 (Two marks if you chose option "3.")

Even though NSAIDs have frequent minor side effects and even though these drugs all too often have serious side effects (ulcers, hemorrhaging, kidney failure, high blood pressure, etc.) and even though the indication for these drugs is often dubious, doctors still prescribe these drugs very liberally. Why?

1. doctors often feel pressured by patients for a prescription
2. it takes a lot less time to fill out a prescription than to give an explanation and reassurance
3. the drug companies make their products sound so-o-o-o good!
4. it makes doctors feel more useful if they can give out a prescription in attempts to relieve their patients' suffering (even when the prescription isn't likely to help)
5. all of the above

Answer: 5. True story.

There are many types of NSAID drugs available. This simple fact tells us that:

1. there must be a lot of people with arthritis
2. one NSAID is not *the* best one
3. with each new addition it is yet one more thing for doctors to have a hard time keeping up with
4. all of the above

Answer: 4.

Ever wonder how your doctor decides which prescription he or she gives you? Well, I'll tell you. Your doctor keeps a close eye on the medical literature, speaks to colleagues, and attends regular lectures, which serve to keep him or her abreast of the state of the art of drug therapy. *Wouldn't it be nice* ... (apologies to the Beach Boys).

Really want to know how your doctor decides?

Well, to be fair many doctors do indeed make their decisions for all the right, scientific reasons. But (there had to be a but didn't there?) there are significant numbers of physicians whose main decision-making arises from the impact of advertising by drug companies.

It continually amazes me how often the newest drug on the block is prescribed when there are often many older, equally effective drugs with a much longer track record for both safety and efficacy. But these older drugs are usually generically available and hence less profitable for the drug companies so they don't promote them. And doctors often get suckered in by multi-million dollar sales pitches for the "new and improved" product.

The advertising is quite fascinating to follow. First the drug companies play peak-a-boo with stark ads in the medical journals usually limited to an almost blank page with a striking caption such as "Coming soon ... A new breakthrough from Flotsam & Jetsam Pharmaceuticals." Just to whet your appetite, I guess.

That goes on for a few months following which, excitement at a fever pitch (?), the journals will have five-page spreads full of dramatic photos, captivating headlines, and striking statements about the "proven efficacy" of Drug X.

Simultaneous to this, pharmaceutical company representatives ("drug reps") beat paths to doctors' offices promoting the new wonder drug. Why do the physicians bother to hear the sales pitch? Sometimes because they need to get free samples for their less well-off patients and if they take the new drug sample the salesperson will leave samples of the other drugs that the doctor really needs. Sometimes because the salesperson will leave "gifts" behind (invitations to play golf, theatre tickets, hockey tickets, etc.). And sometimes because there do exist physicians who put tremendous value in the "information" imparted by the drug reps.

So I ask you: do you want to be getting the newest drug on the market? Well, if it was to treat a disease for which no other, more effective therapy was available then of course there would be merit to it. But what if the new drug was just one more addition to many other currently available and already proven therapeutic options? Do you want to risk being one of the "case reports" that inevitably enter the literature soon after a drug's release wherein Patient A has been found to be the first one ever to have developed hepatitis (or kidney failure or anemia or whatever) after taking Drug X?

Give me tried and true. I don't want one of my patients to be the subject of the next case report. An old adage given to doctors: "Never be the first one to prescribe a new drug nor the last to stop using an old one."

I routinely used to meet with drug reps and hear their pitch, all the time scoffing to myself at what they had to say. Then one day I realized I was prescribing their drugs. Not because of some landmark medical study in the literature, but because I too had been taken in by their pitch. I didn't think I had, but I was wrong. How arrogant of me to have thought that I would not be influenced by the massive advertising campaigns and well-researched sales promotion techniques that had been choreographed. So I made a decision; not out of principal, but rather because I realized I was not quite so strong-willed as I had thought. Except in exceptional circumstances, I would not meet with the pharmaceutical reps. So far this has helped me make my drug choices for more purely scientific reasons, but now if I could just figure out how to avoid those darn ads in the medical journals.

Not surprisingly, osteoarthritis of weight-bearing joints such as the knees is much more common if you subject these joints to excess weight. So, obesity is a big problem here. Just like it is, though of course for entirely different reasons, when it comes to diseases such as hypertension, diabetes, high cholesterol, and so on. Now when I get asked to see an obese person with sore knees I admit that my initial reaction is not sympathetic. Rather, it is indignant. It shouldn't be, but it is. There you have it. Oh, and by the way, I'll take the liberty of speaking for my silent colleagues and let you know that invariably they feel the same way. (Sure eases my conscience when I spread the guilt around).

This indignance can make it terribly difficult to be empathetic and, as the situation dictates, sympathetic, when what you actually feel is frustration and anger. *What in the world does Mr. Grande think I can do for his knees?! He's three hundred pounds for God's sake. If he lost some weight that would do him a lot more good than any drug I could possibly prescribe.*

There is, however, one thing about obesity for which I will forever praise the heavens. It is responsible for my marriage.

I was a resident working on an in-patient ward where severely obese patients were being treated with very strict calorie restriction. The official title was the "metabolic ward." Some residents unkindly called it the "fat farm." One day, another resident who I knew only passingly came out of a patient's room muttering and, to my amazement (until now she had always been exceptionally proper — which probably explains why I hadn't gotten to know her better), she was swearing.

"Shit! Boy that pisses me off."

"What? What did you say? Heather, I can't believe you actually talk like that! What's wrong?" I asked her. I was quite incredulous.

"You know why these people are in hospital, right?" she asked rhetorically. "Well, I just sat down on this lady's bed to do a blood gas (*a test where blood is taken from an artery in the wrist*) and the bed crunched.

Crunched! I pulled down the sheet and there must have been a dozen bags of potato chips there. Why the hell are we spending money and time keeping people in the hospital to lose weight if they don't even follow their diet? And you know what really bugs me," she went on, "I couldn't get the f-ing blood gas because her wrist was so large I couldn't even find the artery."

I knew it was love. Heather and I went down to the cafeteria to commiserate and, as they say, the rest is history.

One of my pet peeves is the term "rheumatism." It is one of those pseudo-scientific non-medical terms that masquerades as medicalese. It does not really mean arthritis. It does not really mean muscle pain. Or back pain. Or anything else for that matter. It is a useless word. Get the idea?

That said, I was obviously being a bit too pedantic when, upon being asked by a patient if she was suffering from rheumatism, I went into a long-winded explanation as to more appropriate terms to describe her illness. It therefore served me right when the patient asked why it was then that sitting on my bookshelf was a very current issue of a journal adorned in large letters with the title "Arthritis and Rheumatism." Oops.

Being pontifical with patients is a skill rapidly acquired by most doctors. Indeed, it is bred by circumstances wherein sick people are understandably going to defer to the person they perceive to have the power to make them better. Unfortunately, given the inherent dynamics in this interchange, there is a tendency amongst physicians to forget where the line is drawn separating pertinent inquiries from superfluous or, at times, intrusive ones.

I first became aware of this in first year medical school when, to demonstrate how to obtain a history, the instructor brought a patient into the lecture hall to be questioned by the students. The man, an engineer of considerable intelligence and patience, took our questions in stride as we asked him about his recent problem with abdominal pain. He told us what the pain had felt like, what it was like to undergo surgery, and so on. After an hour or so, the session came to a conclusion.

The moderator asked us if we had found it a useful exercise and we assured him we had. Then the moderator turned to the patient and asked him if he had anything further to tell us. He did. And what he said gave us pause to think. And indeed, I still think about it.

"You are medical students. Soon you are going to be physicians. There isn't going to be anybody looking over your shoulder to tell you when you are doing something right or wrong. You've asked me a lot of questions today. But do you know *why* you've asked all those things? Did it really matter that my mother abandoned us when I was a kid? Or that I've been having some financial troubles? You have got to know *why* you ask the questions you do. Don't ask them just because you're *curious*. Make sure you have a reason."

That was years ago. But I still remember his advice and try to follow it. There are times, however, that I fail.

I was talking to a patient a while back and asked her, as is customary, if there was any pertinent family history of medical disorders. She told me, like so many patients do, that she was adopted. In this case, however, she then went on to tell me that she had tracked down her birth mother and thus, knew that there was nothing salient in the medical background. I was fascinated by her story. I had never known any adopted individuals that had met up with a birth parent. *What was it like meeting her?* I asked. *Stressful? Intriguing? Were you excited? Disappointed with what she was like? Did she look like you?* After a while I realized that my patient was beginning to look frustrated. *Oh hell, I* thought, *I've crossed the line.* My questions had transgressed that boundary between the medically necessary (and politely sociable) and the prying. So hard to always strike the right balance, being so careful not to say the wrong thing, whilst at the same time not wanting to come across as disinterested or stilted.

People think of arthritis as being a disease of the joints. It almost always comes as a surprise to patients when they hear that many forms of arthritis can also affect:

1. the penis
2. the eyes
3. the nails
4. all of the above

Answer: 4. And indeed virtually every other organ. For example, people with lupus (systemic lupus erythematosis) can get kidney failure and those with rheumatoid arthritis can get inflammation of the lungs. Far from being just pains in the joints, arthritis can wreck havoc on the whole body.

John Rames was a fifty-year-old business consultant whose job frequently took him to various cities across the continent. One day, he came to the emergency department with an acutely sore and swollen left knee. He felt completely well otherwise. I asked him some questions.

Had he ever had any joint pains in the past? No. (Thus, we were not dealing with a chronic disease process. Osteoarthritis, for example, would typically cause insidiously progressive symptoms, not suddenly onsetting ones.)

Did any other joints bother him? No. (Suggesting, therefore, that we were dealing with a very isolated process, unlike rheumatoid arthritis, which typically would affect a number of joints simultaneously).

Any other symptoms? No. (Making it less likely that he had a generalized arthritis process such as lupus which, for example, might cause pleurisy.)

Any sexual contacts during his travels? Yes. It was not all that unusual for him to engage in casual sexual relations during his trips. (Hence, I wondered about the possibility of a sexually transmitted disease, now more commonly known in medical jargon as an STD, the term "venereal disease" having fallen by the wayside. Which is probably for the best because I never did figure out what exactly venereal meant. Always sounded too much like venial or veal or something.)

STDs are no longer the select few diseases they used to be. Gone is the era when syphilis and gonorrhea were all there was. We now live in an era where sexually transmitted diseases also include:

1. Hepatitis B
2. AIDS
3. genital warts
4. herpes
5. all of the above

Answer: 5. And the list goes on and on.

When I examined Mr. Rames there was very little to find with the exception of his left knee. On examining a joint, the physician evaluates a number of things. Firstly, you look at it. Just look. Always the first step. There is such a temptation to jump right in and feel it, manipulate it, press it, poke it ... you get the idea. You have to keep reminding yourself to start the exam by just looking. Mr. Rames's knee looked puffy, suggesting the presence of fluid within the knee. Manipulating the knee caused him quite a bit of pain. Pressing then releasing the inner ("medial") aspect of the knee caused a fleeting dimpling similar to momentarily indenting a plastic bag filled with water. This is called a positive "bulge sign." It confirmed the presence of fluid within the knee.

At this point there was certainly a lot to go on, but not enough to conclusively establish a diagnosis. People just don't realize how much information comes from this approach. A history. Then a physical. The rest is complementary. The blood tests, urine samples, x-rays, EKGs, and so on are primarily measures to confirm a diagnosis that is thought highly probable based on clinical grounds in and of themselves. An over-reliance on these sorts of tests (not to mention more costly modalities such as C.A.T. and M.R.I. scanning) is generally a waste of time and money.

The next step was to perform:

1. an EKG
2. a chest x-ray
3. a rectal examination
4. an arthrocentesis

Answer: 4. An arthrocentesis is also known as a "joint tap." Very crude, very simple, and very helpful. You swab the skin with some cleaning solution (generally iodine) and insert a needle, without need for anaesthetic, under the knee cap (the "patella"). Once the needle is in you pull back on the plunger of the attached syringe and suck out the fluid from the knee. Sounds painful, but it isn't particularly so. At least that is what my patients tell me. (Have you ever heard of a doctor actually submitting to the things that they do to their patients?)

Mr. Rames's knee was filled with cloudy fluid. Cloudy yellow fluid. There shouldn't have been any fluid at all. That still did not clinch a diagnosis; not yet, but that would come shortly thereafter.

An hour after the joint tap was done an excited call came from the laboratory technologist. "Dr. Blumer, Mr. Rames's knee fluid is loaded with gram negative diplococci!" she told me. Gram negative diplococci. Meaning the stain developed years ago by Dr. Gram was taken up poorly (hence "negative") by twinned (hence "diplo") rounded (hence "cocci") bacteria.

Mr. Rames's had:

1. rheumatoid arthritis
2. gonococcal arthritis (caused by gonorrhea)
3. tuberculous arthritis (caused by tuberculosis)
4. psoriatic arthritis (arthritis associated with psoriasis)

Answer: 2.

He had had intercourse with an infected prostitute. The gonococcus germ had entered his urethra, invaded his blood stream and then took up residence in his left knee. Bizarre as this sounds it is not uncommon. In fact the gonococcus can even take up habitat on the heart valves (a disease called "endocarditis"). Quite a nasty little pest, that gonococcus.

Chapter Nine

WEIGHT GAIN, ANHEDONIA,
AND SEEKING THE TRUTH

Weight gain is at once one of the most simple and yet one of the most difficult problems to assess. Generally speaking, by the time someone seeks out medical help for this it has been quite chronic. Far different from people with chest pain who tend to seek rapid medical attention. Clearly, people appreciate the potential seriousness of chest pain and the comparatively benign nature of weight gain. Benign in the sense of not being immediately life-threatening, but certainly not with regard to the potentially devastating impact on one's long term health.

The majority of obese individuals encountered in day-to-day practice present not specifically because of their obesity, but because of health problems arising as a consequence of it. There are, however, a number of people who do seek medical attention to see if there is some underlying disease to explain their overweight state.

Obesity is commonly caused by "gland problems." This is:

1. true
2. false

Answer: 2. Disease of a "gland" seldom causes obesity. In fact very few diseases even exist that are known to cause obesity.

Lois was a twenty-eight-year-old woman who was referred to me because of weight gain. She had also noticed that her voice had become somewhat horse and that her limb muscles had started to ache.

She likely had:

1. cancer of the larynx (the voicebox)
2. lactose intolerance
3. lead poisoning
4. hypothyroidism (an underactive thyroid gland)

Answer: 4.

In examining a patient suspected to have hypothyroidism there are a group of things to look for. A puffy face. "Bags" under the eyes ("infra-orbital edema"). A slow heart beat. And fascinatingly, hypothyroid patients may lose hair from the outer edges ("lateral margins") of their eyebrows. This occurs because hypothyroidism causes the hair to become brittle and to fall out more readily and hence, when your eyebrows rub on your pillow some hair gets literally rubbed off.

When I interviewed Lois I found out that she had been taking a cholesterol lowering medication for the past couple of years. I was thrilled to be able to tell her she would likely be able to come off this in the very near future.

Why?

1. cholesterol-lowering drugs are toxic in patients with hypothyroidism
2. cholesterol-lowering drugs interact adversely with thyroid hormone supplements
3. hypothyroidism causes high cholesterol
4. woman do not benefit from cholesterol-lowering drugs

Answer: 3. True story. And when such patients are rendered euthyroid (that is, when their thyroid status is normalized), their cholesterol levels often return to normal.

Having hypothyroidism is like putting the whole body into low gear. Everything becomes sluggish. Hair growth, perspiration, the heart rate, the bowels ... all slow down. This is especially apparent when you examine the reflexes. Tap the ankle and the foot flexes normally, but there is a delay in how long it takes for the muscles to relax letting the foot extend back to its normal position. You can also see a similar sort of phenomenon when checking for something called pseudomyotonia. You tap a muscle (typically the tricep area) with a reflex hammer and watch for the time it takes for the muscle to then relax. In hypothyroidism this time is longer than normal.

Because hypothyroidism is so common and because it can present with such nonspecific and sometimes quite nebulous symptoms, doctors have a very low threshold in deciding when to order thyroid blood levels.

Patients who have appropriately-treated hypothyroidism will nonetheless frequently continue to have symptoms attributable to their malfunctioning thyroid. This is:

1. true
2. false

Answer: 2. If the hypothyroidism is treated with the correct dose of thyroid hormone supplementation then all symptoms due to the hypothyroidism will gradually clear. Unfortunately, most people do not realize this and for years to come will blame any fatigue, dry skin, constipation (and obesity!) on their "thyroid condition."

Cushing's Syndrome is one of the very few other diseases that can lead to inexplicable weight gain. In this condition, one has excessive levels of a steroid hormone called cortisol. It has various causes, one of them being a tumour of an adrenal gland. Much more commonly, Cushing's is *iatrogenic* (literally meaning, "something the doctor has caused") arising as a consequence of long term use of steroid pills (usually one called prednisone. Note that this is different from anabolic steroids that some athletes use).

Prednisone is truly a wondrous drug. Tens of thousands of people owe their lives to this drug. It is used to treat diseases as diverse as asthma and lupus. It can help many people with bronchitis, pneumonia, colitis, brain tumours, and is even used to prevent rejection of organ transplants. It is definitely one of the major discoveries in the history of medicine. But like many seemingly wondrous things it comes at a price and, in the case of prednisone, the price is not primarily monetary.

I once had an allergic reaction to a vaccination and I needed to take prednisone for a couple of weeks. Being like most physicians I went down to the local pharmacy to get the drug at cost. (Not fair, I know, but what should I do? Pay more than I have to because it is unjust that well-paid physicians get their drugs at cost yet others who can ill-afford it must pay full price? Maybe so, but I don't think I could bring myself to do that.) Two weeks supply cost $2.50. "Bill," I said to the pharmacist, "that can't be right."

"It is," he told me. "In fact, the plastic container is almost as expensive as the pills themselves." I was dumbstruck. Here was a drug that saved life after life and yet was cheaper than most cold remedies.

When given in small doses and for brief periods of time prednisone has little in the way of side effects. Weight gain tends to be minimal or nonexistent. However, when given in larger doses and for longer periods of time, side effects can be so devastating that taking the drug creates problems worse than the disease that was being treated in the first place. Weight gain, as bad a side effect as it is, is one of the comparatively benign ones.

Other side effects from long-term prednisone use include all of the following *except*:

1. high blood pressure
2. stretch marks ("striae")
3. diabetes
4. cataracts
5. edema
6. osteoporosis
7. mood disturbance
8. anhedonia

Answer: 8.

Anhedonia means:

1. seeking pleasure
2. being unable to obtain pleasure
3. thinning of the hair
4. iron deficiency

Clue: *Annie Hall's* original title was reputed to have been "Anhedonia."

Answer: 2. And if you can trust what you hear about Woody Allen you will know why he would have called a film "Anhedonia." Apparently he got persuaded to change the film's name because it was thought that the peculiar original title would turn people off from going to see the film.

Because chronic prednisone use can have such horrendous side-effects, most doctors dispensing it to a patient for long-term use will tell them in detail what can potentially happen from it. This is definitely the exception to the way that physicians generally behave. In fact, advising patients about possible side effects from most prescription drugs simply does not usually happen. And we have lots of excuses for this inaction; some quite justified, some not.

Excuse number one: If I tell Mr. Singh that Inderal (Propranolol) may make him fatigued it's guaranteed that two days later he's going to call to let me know that, "Gee whiz, doctor. You were right. That pill sure does make me tired."

Excuse number two: If I inform Mrs. O'Leary that the digoxin she needs for her heart failure can potentially cause a life-threatening heart rhythm disorder, she's not very likely to take it even though she needs it.

Excuse number three: Mrs. Steinman has been my patient for fifteen years. She is eighty-five years old and her memory has been failing. She trusts me to use my judgment to select what treatment is best for her. She doesn't want to hear the litany of things that may or may not occur with this or that drug and she wouldn't be able to understand or remember anyhow.

Excuse number four: The list of side effects from Tegretol (carbamazepine) is so long that it takes up two pages in my drug book. I wouldn't even know where to begin to tell Mr. Johansen what it is that could go wrong.

Excuse number five: The drug stores nowadays give detailed handouts to the patients and I'm running late anyway. Mrs. Rodin can get the info from the pharmacist when she picks up her prescription.

The list goes on and on.

The bottom line here is that if you are the patient and if you are interested in your health care then you've got to make a point of asking questions and getting answers. If you want, after the examination has concluded bring in a relative or friend (you know what they say about two heads) so you can both hear what the doctor has to say. And if you do ask questions, make sure that you understand the answers. Even if your doctor is in a rush. Who says the next patient is more important than you? When you are in the office, you should be your doctor's number one priority. Make sure that you get comprehensible explanations not only about your drugs, but about the illness that the doctor is prescribing the drugs for. It's cut and dry. You are the patient. The doctor works for you.

This is clearly a straightforward issue. So much so that I feel both vehement and dogmatic about it. Funny though that when my accountant or my lawyer or, for that matter, my grocer gives me an explanation about something or other, I'm often afraid to ask questions for fear of looking stupid or needlessly delaying them.

Cushing's Syndrome causes a number of physical changes. Typically one gets a rounded facial appearance (a "moon facies"), a lump on the upper back (a "buffalo hump") and a belly that is disproportionately fatter than the limbs (a "lemon on a toothpick" appearance). These things occur because of the actions of cortisol hormone on the body's fat stores mobilizing them from the extremities and depositing them centrally. The skin becomes thinner and more fragile resulting in stretch marks (striae) on the abdomen and bruising on the limbs. The body starts to retain salt and water leading to both high blood pressure and ankle swelling. Not very nice is it? Well, as I said before, this drug saves lives, but at a cost.

There is an old medical saying (well actually I have no idea if it's old or not; sounds like it is anyhow) that a disease may be rare, but for the patient that has it, the frequency is 100 percent. So when I see a patient for a problem such as obesity the onus is on me to make sure they do not have some problem other than simple dietary indiscretion. Which brings up the issue of error in diagnosis.

I wish I was always right. Like most (though definitely not all) physicians, I try my best to stay current and to look after patients properly. But as much as I hate to admit it I do screw up. I do not know a single doctor who has not yet made an incorrect diagnosis, or given the wrong treatment for the right diagnosis, or given the right treatment for the wrong diagnosis or some permutation or combination of these. Why do we physicians get it wrong? Actually I think a better question might be why do we seem to generally get it right (hush, you cynics out there who would dispute even that).

Medicine is a very quickly evolving discipline. It is said that the doubling time of medical knowledge is five years. So what you learn today is old news tomorrow. And out of date soon after that. Couple that with the all-too-obvious ability of humans to err and it does not take too much stretch of the imagination to see why doctors get it wrong. Now that sounds like I am declaring a general amnesty for physicians who mess things up. So then, let me add that I think a lot of mistakes do indeed come from physicians' laziness and, at times, downright incompetence.

Sometimes it is a cascade of errors that takes place. Individually they might not be disastrous, but when taken together they can lead to catastrophe. To illustrate, let me relate the following true-to-life scenario.

A forty-five-year-old man comes to the emergency department. He tells the triage nurse (the nurse doing the initial patient assessment and determining the patient's relative priority for seeing the doctor) that he has a dull, aching chest pain. The nurse finds the patient to look quite comfortable and since the "crisis" room is full anyhow, she puts him in a regular cubicle (problem #1). He is eventually assessed by the overwrought emergency room physician who, feeling pressured because of the number of patients he has yet to see (problem #2), gets quickly frustrated by the patient's vague description of his pain (problem #3), hastily concludes that the patient's pain sounds innocuous and tells the nurse to get an EKG when she has time (problem #4). The doctor gets busy looking after a trauma patient and only gets back to see the patient two hours later (problem #5), at which point he quickly scans the EKG and, not expecting to see anything much (problem #6), surprise, surprise, he does not see anything much (problem #7), thereby having overlooked the subtle but important abnormalities that are, in fact, present. The patient is sent home with a diagnosis of muscular chest pain (problem #8) and advised to see his family doctor the next day, at which point a repeat EKG shows much more severe abnormalities, the patient is admitted to the intensive care unit (more aptly termed the expensive care unit or, heaven forbid, the insensitive care unit) with a diagnosis of acute myocardial infarction (heart attack) and the patient lies in bed wondering how those idiots in the emergency department screwed up. Believe you me, it's easy. And it happens. Indeed, it is said that 10 percent (!!) of all heart attack victims going to the emergency department are misdiagnosed and sent home.

Like cops, physicians are often criticized for "sticking together"; for not condemning their colleagues who have erred even if the mistake was owing to what appears to be glaring incompetence. But if you want to know why doctors almost never publicly criticize one another, the answer lies in the story above, for each and every physician has seen this or similar sorts of disasters and prays that they won't be the next one to screw up. We all know it not only *can* happen to us but, given enough time, it *will* happen to us.

The unfortunate result is that physicians are so hesitant to criticize their colleagues that notoriously bad physicians, those who are unfailingly inept, end up being protected until such time that one of their many blunders leads to either a law suit, or a complaint to their governing body.

As I mentioned earlier, most cases of obesity are not due to any "organic" disease. That is, there is no specific medical illness responsible. It is simply that overweight people:

1. eat too much
2. have sluggish bowels
3. have a slow metabolism

Answer: 1. Granted, there are those individuals whose bodies have become less efficient at burning off calories, but the bottom line remains that if your weight is to remain steady "calories in must equal calories out." If you truly "eat like a bird," it is guaranteed you will not look like a whale. Forgive the comparison, but pictures of drought-stricken regions of Africa graphically attest to this fact.

Unfortunately, people do not like to hear this. I used to try to explain to my overweight patients the dynamics of calorie consumption versus expenditure. I got nowhere. Or even worse, patients got mad at me for suggesting that they were over-eating. I am somewhat embarrassed to admit that I had to learn what should have been obvious to me at the outset: people don't want to be told the things they choose not to believe or feel they have no control over. It just frustrates or angers them. I should have known this. If someone is convinced they eat "nothing" but are still unable to lose weight they do not want to be told that they are wrong; that they cannot possibly be "eating nothing."

It was only when reading an article on a totally unrelated medical topic that I came across the term which I now, when seeing such patients, keep repeating to myself as if it were a mantra. "A sympathetic hearing." People just want a sympathetic hearing. It is so self-evident that I could kick myself for not having realized this obvious truism long ago.

People do not want to be berated, lectured to, admonished about or in any other way told how their eating habits, pure and simple, are responsible for their being overweight. "Calories in = calories out" belongs in the lecture hall, not the doctor's office. To be reassured there is nothing seriously wrong with them is nice, but not enough. They don't feel like they are misbehaving, or overeating, or underexercising. Life *just isn't being fair* to them. And I tell them so. And they nod. *Someone understands.* I didn't used to, but I do now. I cannot prescribe any medication to help them, but a bit of empathy leaves them feeling satisfied nonetheless. For me, though, I feel far less satisfied. A little charade has simply been played out. I know that they are simply overeating. Indeed, studies have confirmed that overweight patients uniformly underestimate their food intake. But people do not want either to hear this or to believe it. So I acquiesce. And feel like I have accomplished little.

Chapter Ten

DIARRHEA, CONSTIPATION, SILVER PATIENTS,
AND SCARY INTERNS

People and their bowels amaze me. I'm not sure which amazes me the most, but certainly the two together do. People can have excruciating difficulty in describing their chest pains or their headaches or their abdominal pains, but invariably details of their stools are recounted with precision. Soft or hard. Loose or formed. Small or large. Twice a day or twice a year. This meticulous recalling of one's bowel habits is all for the better in helping establish a diagnosis. Helpful, that is, if the patient has come because of a bowel problem. But when they are being seen for some totally unrelated problem, a precise recounting of their stooling pattern can be, ahem, a pain in the butt.

This particularly strikes home when looking after very ill patients in the intensive care unit. More than once (a lot more than once!) I've had patients in hospital with a heart attack who, when I ask them how they are feeling tell me not about their severe chest pain, nor their breathlessness, but rather about the fact that they have not had a bowel movement in two days. In some ways it is a good sign that, despite having just had a heart attack, they should feel well enough to worry about their bowels. I used to think this was a cultural phenomenon. And so it is — it affects every culture on earth.

Speaking about intensive care units reminds me of what surely must be the quintessential example of inserting one's lowermost appendage into one's oral cavity. Dr. Bearnam, a famous cardiologist in a well-known teaching hospital, was making rounds with the house-staff (interns, residents, etc.). We went into the room of an elderly man by the name of Abramson. He was recovering from a heart attack.

"So Ian, how is Mr. Abramson doing?" Dr. Bearnam asked.

"Very well sir," I answered. "He's now three days post infarct and hasn't had any complications. I'm hoping to get him out of bed into a chair today."

"Three days post infarct. And you haven't had him up walking yet?! Come on Ian, what are you waiting for?" he said as he pulled down the bedsheets exposing Mr. Abramson's chest, belly, genitalia, thighs, and stumps. Double amputee.

"Shit," Dr. Bearnam muttered as he turned around and walked out of the room.

Dr. Bearnam was one of those rare people that once you've met you never, ever forget. (I'm sure Mr. Abramson could vouch for that). Anecdotes concerning him are legion.

He did not like to deal with stupid people. Bad enough, in his opinion, to deal with stupid patients (and he was, to be fair, truly brilliant and perhaps for that reason tended to think of most people as stupid), but to have to deal with stupid doctors, well, that was just too much.

We were on ward rounds (the traditional circuit of the ward made by physicians) when we stopped outside a patient's door. "So John, tell me about this patient," Dr. Bearnam said.

"He's a sixty-year-old man who has had a fever for three days. His exam was unremarkable. I put him on antibiotic therapy with Ancef and Tobra."

"Why did you do that?" Dr. B. asked

"Because he had a fever," John answered.

Uh, oh, I thought to myself. *Now he's done it.*

"John, you putz. How the hell do *you* treat a fever? I treat it with Tylenol."

"But, but," John stammered when Dr. B interrupted him.

"What you *mean* John is that you thought the patient had a bacterial infection and so you put him on antibiotics to treat *that; not* his fever. Right? Right?!"

"Yeah. I mean yes. Of course."

"So say it next time. You got that?!"

Dr. B did not like John. I think the feeling was mutual.

Though he could be unbelievably cruel to his house staff, all of us (even those who were on the receiving end of his wrath) did recognize

Dr. Bearnam's great ability to teach. Whether he was giving a classroom lecture or a hallway denunciation, he did truly help us to develop our clinical skills. "Be consistent," had to be his favourite motto. "If you make the wrong diagnosis, that may be excusable so long as you at least gave the treatment indicated for that (wrong) diagnosis. Don't compound your error by making a wrong diagnosis then not being true to your premise."

He was also renowned as being supportive of his house staff so long as they were straight with him. One day, a fellow resident of mine was in the emerg looking after a patient having a heart attack. In order to lessen the risk of a heart rhythm disorder, he gave her an intravenous medication. But ten times the recommended dose. The patient had an epileptic seizure as a result. The resident was devastated. He was a conscientious, thoughtful, and caring person who had just made a terrible mistake. In tears, he immediately went to Dr. Bearnam's office and told him what he had done. Expecting shouts and condemnation, he cowered in fear and guilt. Instead, he felt a fatherly arm around his shoulder. "Leon, you screwed up. You really screwed up. But you obviously recognize it and you haven't tried to hide from your mistake. And I'm sure you'll never make that mistake again. Now go back to work."

Fortunately the patient did not suffer any permanent injury. Leon explained to her what he had done and she held no grudge against him. Nonetheless, to this day Leon talks about his horror over the incident. (And I suspect the patient does too).

How many people realize just how often mistakes are made by their doctors? Not many, I'd wager. Because if you knew you would tread in fear every time you went to see a doctor or were admitted to hospital. Especially if it was a teaching hospital (though, of course, in teaching hospitals they say the same about community hospitals).

As interns and residents, medical school having only recently been completed, you don't know a hell of a lot and it is very easy to mess up. Very easy. People think that if you are a patient in an urban, university-affiliated teaching hospital, then you have "the best" doctors around. Think again. Sure, most (but not by any stretch of the imagination, all) of the staff physicians may have impressive academic credentials and indeed, may be the best in their field. But did you know that the majority of the day (and all of the night) the doctors looking after you — assessing your chest pain, treating your bleeding and, I tell you the truth, running the cardiac arrests — are the most junior physicians in the place?

I remember my very first day as an intern. I was on call at a large cancer hospital. It was about two in the morning as I made my way down a long, dim corridor en route to see a patient. He'd taken a sudden turn for the worse and the nurses wondered if he was going into shock. As I strode along I was feeling very self-important. I was *the* doctor on call. What a trip. Then it hit me like a ton of bricks. I sure was the doctor on call. In fact I was the *only* doctor in the entire hospital. And this was my very first day as a physician. Like, one moment here: what's wrong with this picture? The responsibility was far beyond my capabilities. And I do not say that out of modesty. I was a good intern, but the responsibility was far beyond *any* intern's capabilities.

Lest you think I am being a bit too melodramatic here, let me relate another incident to you.

A twenty-five-year-old second-year medical resident was making his ward rounds in the ICU He was feeling rotten. Having come down with infectious mononucleosis ("mono"), he should have been home in bed, but he knew if he wasn't working one of his already overburdened colleagues would have even more to do. So he was trying his best to look after his patients. But, having just left a patient's bedside, he suddenly felt something "give" in his belly and he collapsed onto the floor. Rushed to the operating room he was found to have ruptured his spleen.

After being initially stable, that night things started to go downhill. His blood pressure fell. His kidneys started producing less urine. The nurse on duty became concerned and summoned the intern on call. Having examined the patient, the intern looked at the patient and said; "looks like you're retaining too much fluid; I'll give you some Lasix (a diuretic)."

The patient, lying semi-stuporous in bed, drowsy from low blood pressure, sensorium further clouded by morphine, could barely understand what the intern was saying.

"Okay, okay, whatever you say," he mumbled. Then, as he lay there, he started to mull things over. Something wasn't right. *Kidneys not working. Low blood pressure. A diuretic? Huh? Is that right? No, that doesn't sound right. No. Hey wait a second here. What I need is fluids, not diuretics.*

The patient struggled into consciousness. He knew he would be dead if he didn't. "Sam, stop! Not diuretics. I've probably bled. Give me fluids. Get the surgeon to come in."

"You think so?" Sam answered. "Okay, I'll give her a call."

Thankfully, Sam did get her to come in. And she quickly sorted things out and gave the patient the life-saving transfusion that he had needed all along. It was a close call. Any closer and you wouldn't be reading this book right now.

Constipation is far and away the most frequent bowel complaint and, as with virtually any other symptom, what you tell the doctor is the key to establishing a diagnosis.

Mr. Thomas was a seventy-year-old man who came to see me

because of some bowel troubles. He had generally been in good health, but over the past six months he had become increasingly constipated.

The best thing to do at this stage would be to:

1. tell Mr. Thomas that constipation is inevitable with aging — he needn't worry
2. tell Mr. Thomas nothing
3. send Mr. Thomas for a barium enema
4. send Mr. Thomas for thyroid tests

Answer: 2. Remember what I said earlier in this book. History, history, history. Do not jump to conclusions. Get as much information from the patient as you can before you do anything else. Otherwise you will end up wasting time and sending patients for needless tests. When taking a history it is the time to listen, not to tell.

Mr. Thomas related how he had never before been constipated. He had also noticed that the calibre of his stools had narrowed. And he saw a bit of blood with the stool.

Important things to determine about the blood he saw include all of the following *except*:

1. was it mixed in with the stool
2. was it coating the stool
3. had he eaten red meat a day or two before he noticed the blood
4. was it in the toilet water also

Answer: 3. Red meat can give false-positive readings when testing stools for occult blood (i.e. microscopic levels of blood) but does not cause visible blood in the stool. Blood coating the stool suggests a problem in the rectum or anus. Blood mixed in with the stool suggests a lesion more internally.

Mr. Thomas's blood was on the outside of the stool, streaking it.

His having noticed smaller calibre stools suggests a possible problem in which *two* areas?

1. stomach
2. small bowel
3. large bowel
4. rectum

Answer: 3 and 4.

The rest of the history was unremarkable as was the physical examination. A subsequent barium enema (an x-ray of the large bowel) was normal.

The next step would be to:

1. do a sigmoidoscopy (that is, put a scope up his backside to look directly at the rectum)
2. reassure the patient that there is nothing seriously amiss and he should just live with his problem
3. do thyroid tests
4. send the patient for a barium x-ray of the stomach (an "upper g.i.")

Answer: 1. Patients and physicians alike are often not aware of the fact that the rectum is not well seen on a barium enema. When doing a barium enema, a balloon tipped nozzle is inserted into the rectum and inflated. The barium goes through the nozzle and into the large bowel. Barium in the large bowel shows up on the x-ray. The rectum itself however is filled with the balloon and thus not with the barium. Thus, it is impossible to know if there is a problem there or not unless you look directly at the rectum with a scope. People have died from rectal cancer that would have been picked up at a curable stage if only their doctors had known that simple fact.

I did a sigmoidoscopy on Mr. Thomas and indeed he had a cancer of the rectum. It was the physical effect of the cancer narrowing the rectum that caused the stools to be narrow and the patient to feel constipated.

Sometimes what starts out as relatively innocuous constipation sets into motion (sorry, couldn't resist) a vicious cycle of worsening constipation. This arises when someone having mild constipation starts to use strong ("irritant") laxatives which, unlike fibre, act directly on the bowel wall to stimulate it. This initially gives good results, but, with time, the bowel gets resistant to the laxative's effects and constipation recurs. People then increase the dose of the laxative or get a stronger one following which they will have temporary improvement followed by worsening. More laxative. Improvement then worsening. And so on. Eventually the bowel gets so "lazy" that intractable, unremitting constipation is present.

I remember the first time a patient told me this type of story. To make sure nothing more sinister was going on I performed a sigmoidoscopy.

Sigmoidoscopy derives its name from the *sigmoid* ("S shaped") colon and the *scope* used to look at it. The conventional sigmoidoscope is a foot-long, straight piece of rigid metal. S-shaped colon *plus* rigid straight scope *equals* people not liking this procedure very much. Should you ever need one you may take heart though; flexible scopes are gradually replacing the rigid kind.

Upon looking into the patient's bowel I observed the startling presence of a dark brown colour. Seriously. No, not brown stool. It was the lining of the bowel which was dark brown. Normally it is pink. This bowel looked deeply suntanned. I did not think it very likely that he had been suntanning his rectum. (Although, having said that, it is actually quite amazing what people do to their rectums. I remember one patient who sheepishly came hobbling into the emergency department saying that he was having rectal pain. An x-ray showed an obstruction. A sigmoidoscopy showed a jar of pickles. And if you have ever wondered if the straight-faced doctor dealing with such a patient then goes into the doctors' lounge and laughs hysterically as he relates the story to his colleagues, you need wonder no more. He does.)

A dark brown discolouration to the lining of the bowel suggests:

1. melanosis coli
2. milk allergy
3. ulcerative colitis
4. Crohn's Disease

Answer: 1. Melanosis coli is a condition of increased pigmentation of the bowel and is a surefire sign of laxative abuse.

Suntanned bowels reminds me of my silver-skinned patient. An elderly woman had come to the hospital because of pneumonia. I went into her room her and was astounded when I cast my eyes upon her silver-coloured face. It was truly silver. Later on, as I presented her case to my fellow interns and residents I could see their disbelieving looks as I recounted my visit with the sterling lady. I took them to meet her and they too came out shaking their heads in disbelief. We did not have a clue as to what was causing this. We excitedly called our senior staff physician to the ward so that we might relate this fascinating case.

I carefully studied his face as I told him about the patient. He looked at me with a bemused expression. I couldn't tell if this represented scepticism or condescension. What it was not was awe at my clinical acumen.

After I finished presenting he smiled paternalistically and asked me whether I had obtained a complete history from her. I assuredly had, I told him.

"Are you certain?" he asked.

"Yes, I'm certain," I said, feeling increasingly uncertain.

"Did you ask about her nose drops?"

"Huh?"

"About her nose drops." he patiently repeated.

"No; should I have?" I asked. Must have sounded brilliant.

"Why of course you should have. This is obviously a case of":

1. jeweller's coryza
2. watchmaker's rhinitis
3. plumbism
4. argyria

Answer: 4.

Of course. Now if only I knew what in the world argyria was. He explained that it was the depositing of silver salts in the skin after absorption from the lining of the nose. How did it get into the nose? From silver-containing nose drops which used to be dispensed. From that experience I learned two things: what argyria was, and how more experience could sure make you look smarter.

Most cases of acute diarrhea are pretty straightforward. Typically this occurs without any other major symptoms and the rest of the family is often simultaneously affected. It usually goes away within a day or two and indeed most people wouldn't even bother to see a doctor.

Such diarrhea is generally due to:

1. viral gastroenteritis
2. food poisoning
3. lactose intolerance
4. peptic ulcer disease

Answer: 1.

Another common cause of diarrhea is food poisoning. The bacteria that most commonly causes food poisoning is:

1. stretococcus

   2. claustidium
   3. legonella
   4. salmonella

Answer: 4.

I remember being over for a barbecue at my brother's house when I noticed him taking the hamburgers off the grill. "STOP!" I yelled when I saw him about to put them back on the same plate that he had used for the raw burgers.

He thought I had gone off the deep end, but I am pleased to report that he was wrong. Both about my reaction and more importantly about his use of the plate. Salmonella bacteria are typically present in raw meat and thus would have been on the plate that had held the uncooked hamburgers. These germs would have been just thrilled to take up residence on the cooked meat and then inside our insides.

Food poisoning due to salmonella often causes bad enough diarrhea that people do seek medical attention. Unfortunately, what then often happens is that a well-meaning doctor places the patient on an antibiotic.

That is unfortunate because:

   1. salmonella should never be treated with antibiotics
   2. salmonella should first be treated with anti-diarrheal agents
   3. antibiotics can prolong salmonella infection
   4. antibiotics should never be used to treat bowel disease

Answer: 3. When antibiotics are given to treat salmonella gastroenteritis, the treatment can in fact prolong infection by inducing a chronic carrier state (that is, causing prolonged retention of the germ in our bodies). It is, therefore, more appropriate to obtain stool cultures and to withhold antibiotics until one is sure that a trial of careful observation has failed to cure the patient. The exception to this rule is when dealing with someone who is clearly very ill with high fevers, severe bloody diarrhea and so on, in which case the institution of antibiotics pending the culture results is indeed quite appropriate.

Treating salmonella when it would be best to not treat it at all is a good example of physicians doing more harm than good. Which we do commonly, albeit with the best of intentions.

As medical students we were taught what our predecessors had also been taught for millennia before us: "primum non nocere."

Above all, do no harm. This, we were told, was one of those rare statements of wisdom at its purest. They were right. This is certainly pure: pure crap. Any doctor prescribing any drug or performing any surgery for any disease knows that there is no way to be sure that you "do no harm." Unexpected side effects from drugs and unexpected complications from surgery do happen. Often. Nonetheless, it still is a good reminder to us to at least think before we leap, or in this case, before we prescribe.

Persisting diarrhea, when associated with weight loss, is a major concern. Tell your doctor you've had diarrhea for the past two months and you've lost twenty pounds and just watch his or her eyes open wide, brows furrow, look intensify ... if not then you have either got a doctor with a very practised demeanour of neutrality or a doctor that should not be your (or anyone else's) doctor.

One cause of persisting diarrhea with weight loss is cancer. Another is malabsorption. In the latter condition you can be eating very well, but all for nought since the nutrients are not getting absorbed from the bowel into the bloodstream.

If you are malabsorbing, your stools will often:

1. float
2. sink

Answer: 1. Fat is more buoyant than water. And if you are malabsorbing that which you eat that would include your fat intake.

If you are malabsorbing you had better get a good toilet brush. This is:

1. true
2. false

Answer: 1. Fat-rich stools stick to the bowl. Tenaciously.

If you are malabsorbing your family will soon let you know they think you have a problem. This is:

1. true
2. false

Answer: 1. And not necessarily because they notice you losing weight. Fatty stools stink. Not just any kind of stink. A God-awful stink. If you don't live alone, you won't suffer alone.

People often think that doctors must feel ill at ease dealing with things like stool, rectal examinations and the like. In fact, that is rarely the case. As bowel specialists say, "it may be shit to you, but it's bread and butter to me."

Chapter Eleven

WEAK AND DIZZY;
OH DOCTOR I'M SO WEAK AND DIZZY

"Weak and dizzy. Oh doctor, I'm *so* weak and dizzy."

Master that simple phrase and you will have developed ultimate power over your doctor. You will leave him or her in a cold sweat, knees trembling and heart pounding. Your doctor will be putty in your hands. For nothing, but nothing is so intimidating to a physician than to have to deal with this combination of symptoms. Either symptom alone does not bestow such power: it has to be both together. And if you happen to be frail and elderly then you may as well just get out a broom and dustpan and sweep the doctor's remains off the floor.

Dorothy Levy was an eighty-five-year-old, mentally bright but physically frail woman who lived on her own. One evening her son repeatedly telephoned her, but there was no answer. Becoming alarmed he went to her apartment, let himself in and found her on the bathroom floor. An ambulance was summoned and she was brought to the emergency department. The emergency room physician heard the story, briefly examined the patient and asked the nurse to "get the internist on call to see the patient."

The "internist on call" (feeling very much like the "intern on call") dutifully came to the emergency department feeling suitably ticked off that the emergency room doctor had not so much as even attempted to try to sort out the basics of the patient's story. He reviewed the nurse's observations and entered the patient's room.

"Mrs. Levy, I'm Dr. Blumer. I'm on call for internal medicine this evening. The emergency room doctor ... no, no Mrs. Levy I'm not an intern, I'm an internist — I do *internal* medicine. Anyhow, Mrs. Levy I've been asked to come see you. I understand you had a fall. Can you tell me about it? You can't? Well, what *do* you remember about it? Not much, eh? I see. Um, do you remember feeling dizzy before you fell? Oh, you're always dizzy. Ah, did you feel like you might pass out? Oh you were 'just dizzy.' Well, did it feel like the room was spinning? No, just dizzy. Did it feel like your vision was going dark? No. Just dizzy. I see. I see."

Getting nowhere at lightening speed, I decided to try a different tack. "Mrs. Levy, try describing what it was like without using the word dizzy?" (an old but useful trick to get additional history when all seems lost). "You can't? Oh. Oh." Deep sigh. I had exhausted my repertoire.

So much for the "history of the present illness" as it is called. Perhaps I would glean more information by obtaining a "systems review." This is the process of inquiring about the other systems of the body not directly involving the apparently diseased organ.

"Any problems with your hearing, Mrs. Levy?" I asked.

"Oh, you wear hearing aids. What's that ... oh I see, you are supposed to but you don't because of the whistling noise. Do you have problems with your vision? Uhuh, two cataracts. Yes, yes, that must make navigating difficult. That cane, Mrs. Levy, is it yours? Oh I see, osteoarthritis of your right hip. You limp. Mrs. Levy when I move your big toe like this can you tell me, is it pointing up or down? You can't tell? Okay. Mrs. Levy, what's that you say, I'm sorry I missed it? A stroke. When? Last year. Uhuh. Uhuh. Yes, I see..." And so it goes.

Why do you think I would have moved the patient's toe up and down?

1. to determine if she was demented
2. to assess proprioception
3. to see if she was paying attention
4. to check her circulation

Answer: 2.

What is proprioception?

1. an awareness of prions
2. a form of contraception
3. similar to extra-sensory perception
4. an awareness of the position of the body

Answer: 4. This is important in assessing dizziness or balance problems because you need to have an awareness of your body position relative to your surroundings in order to maintain balance.

Why might it be worthwhile to see if this patient could feel a vibrating tuning fork placed against her great toe?

1. to see if she had a sense of humour
2. to impress her with the fact that doctors can think up all sorts of bizarre tests
3. to test her dorsal columns
4. to test her pyramidal tract

Answer: 3. Now if you knew this answer you have probably studied physiology somewhere along the way. If you simply guessed right then you get double points and a pat on the back — you'd be a great doctor.

What in the world are dorsal columns?

1. those tall things supporting the Parthenon
2. the back fins on great white sharks
3. a bundle of nerves going up the back part (dorsum) of the spinal cord that carry messages about position and vibration sense to the brain

Answer: 3. The reason to do vibration sense testing lies in the fact that the nerves that carry messages about vibration are the same ones that carry impulses about position sense so if there is a significant defect in the one there typically is a defect in the other.

"Why is this woman dizzy?" the nurse asks after I leave Mrs. Levy's room. I start to explain, but I quickly lose her interest. Simple answers. That's what we all want. Doctors, nurses, patients, relatives. We all want simple, concise, straightforward answers. But for Mrs. Levy and the millions of patients like her there are no simple, concise, straightforward answers. If Mrs. Levy's problem was just failing eyesight she would likely get by. Were it just some arthritis in her hip she would likely cope. Were it just a balance defect she would probably manage. But, like many elderly individuals, it was a myriad of things all at once; so-called "multiple-sensory-deficit syndrome." Failing hearing, eyesight and balance in a frail elderly woman with arthritis in her hips ... any wonder she was "weak and dizzy?"

Thankfully, most cases of dizziness are not quite so complex. Some examples ...

A forty-year-old woman presented to her doctor with recurring bouts of dizziness. They had been present on and off for the past two years. An attack would be characterized by a suddenly onsetting, spinning sensation like she had experienced as a child when she would spin around and around on the front lawn. She had also recently noticed ringing ("tinnitus") in her ears. And, most worrisome of all, she had become aware of some hearing loss.

Diagnosis?

    1. benign positional vertigo
    2. Meniere's disease
    3. brain tumour
    4. labrynthitis

Answer: 2. Meniere's disease. This is an inner ear condition of uncertain cause, inconsistent response to treatment and variable prognosis. Hey, sounds like much of medicine.

A twenty-year-old male roofer tumbled from a ten foot high roof landing on an asphalt driveway. Miraculously, he did not sustain any life-threatening injuries, but he did hit his head hard enough to briefly lose consciousness. He was taken to hospital, held overnight for observation then released. Shortly thereafter, he began experiencing headaches, had difficulty concentrating, and he started to feel dizzy. Not a spinning feeling; just a sensation of unsteadiness. He was not falling or fainting. His examination was normal as were all investigations.

Diagnosis?

    1. post-concussive syndrome
    2. benign positional vertigo
    3. compensation neuroses
    4. malingering

Answer: 1. Post-concussive syndrome. This is, in fact, quite a common problem after a head injury severe enough to have caused loss of consciousness. A post-concussive syndrome can persist for months and can be quite disabling. (By the way, do not ever ask your doctor exactly how common is "common." We need some vagueries. Actually, quite a few. A study was done asking doctors to quantitate what was meant by terms such as "commonly," "not uncommonly," "frequently," "very frequently," and "almost always." The only thing the answers had in common was constant variety — common was one half the time to one physician, 90 percent of the time to another).

A sixty-five-year-old man had a heart attack three months ago. After an initially uneventful recovery he then began having palpitations and dizzy spells. He would be standing, not doing very much, when all of a sudden he would notice his vision suddenly darkening. Next thing he knew, he would find himself lying on the ground. A few times he passed right out.

Most likely diagnosis?

1. "simple" faints
2. shock
3. cardiac rhythm disorder
4. pulmonary emboli (blood clots in the lung)

Answer: 3. He was almost certainly experiencing bouts of a disordered heart rhythm. When the heart is damaged in a heart attack sometimes the injured tissue becomes electrically unstable and triggers abnormal heart beats. If these occur in rapid succession the blood pressure falls, the brain does not get enough oxygen and fainting ensues.

In many cases, despite taking a careful history (there really should be no other type, should there?) and doing a thorough examination (truly thorough would take about four hours, but for all intents and purposes ten to fifteen minutes is plenty), the cause of someone's dizziness remains unclear. This typically leads to numerous tests which equally typically come back normal. And that leads to my next question.

Chronic dizziness with normal investigations is usually due to:

1. an acoustic neuroma (a tumour of the nerve that connects the ear to the brain)
2. a tumour of the cerebellum (the area of the brain controlling position and co-ordination)

3. anxiety or stress
4. a perforated eardrum

Answer: 3.

Doctors typically deem such a cause "functional." You might recall this term from earlier chapters when it was used in relation to other symptoms. I sort of like the word "functional." It's vague enough that patients hearing it are unlikely to take offence. Yet it's specific enough that doctors uniformly know exactly what is meant by its use. Medical jargon is replete with such euphemisms. Particularly colourful are those used to describe patients who are, to put it gently, not Mensa candidates. Supratentorial emphysema, betz cell anemia, and monosynapsia are just a sampling. Believe me when I tell you that these are not complimentary terms.

"Functional" patients often believe they have something terribly wrong despite all evidence to the contrary. And I must admit it can be very tiresome to hear such patients complain over and over and over about the same symptoms. It's quite a challenge to have them come to understand that you really, truly, honestly do believe they are suffering. To them, being told there is nothing seriously wrong is interpreted as a denial of their symptoms. Sometimes the vehemence with which they relate their woes would make one think their lives had come to a complete standstill. Yet they have often carried on any and all activities without difficulty. I finally learned how to use this crucial piece of information to both my patients' and my own advantage.

A patient has terrible dizziness. Yet the examination is normal as are a battery of different tests. The patient has been reassured, but continues to complain bitterly about how dizziness is wrecking his life. I haven't been able to help him at all. Repeated attempts at reassurance have not worked. So, I pull out my secret weapon (well, I guess not so secret from now on).

"With your dizziness being so bad, I guess you must have had to stop driving?" I ask, trying my absolute best to sound neutral.

"Oh no, I can still drive," comes the quick reply.

Then, you see the light turn on. He realizes his licence might be in jeopardy if he has severe, unremitting dizziness. And at the same time he recognizes that in fact he has no problem driving. So it dawns on him that he should be minimizing the problem, accepting that it is there but clearly not incapacitating, and finally getting on with life.

There is, however, a corollary to this; when the occasional patient responds in the affirmative — yes indeed they have given up driving. And just when I had been convinced that their problem was entirely functional. "Now what have I missed?" I ask myself.

Chapter Twelve

SHORTNESS OF BREATH, CHOOSING YOUR
POISON, AND USING A CAGE

There are few symptoms more terrifying than feeling short of breath, being "unable to get enough air in," or in medical parlance, suffering from "dyspnea."

A common cause of shortness of breath is asthma. During asthma attacks the airways become narrowed and this makes it more difficult to get air into or out of the lungs. Asthma attacks can range from the very mild to the very fatal.

A common trigger of asthma attacks is:

1. food allergy
2. a cold
3. stress
4. none of the above

Answer: 2. Upper respiratory tract infections (for example; sinusitis or a cold) are very common precipitating factors. Other triggers include exposure to allergens (examples including dust mites, mould, or animal hair) or to respiratory irritants (such as smoke or smog to name but a few).

When people die from asthma attacks it is often because:

1. no medicine will work in very severe cases
2. they do not seek medical attention fast enough
3. they have an allergic reaction to their drugs
4. none of the above

Answer: 2. When people die from asthma, it is often retrospectively determined that their symptoms had been progressively worsening over the preceding weeks, for which they had been taking escalating doses of their medications. It used to be thought that the medicines themselves had been responsible for the fatal outcomes, but it is now recognized that it was a failure to seek timely medical attention that was responsible, not the drugs. This somewhat insidious course is in marked contrast to highly allergic asthmatics whose attacks can take on life-threatening proportions an instant after exposure to certain stimuli.

Ventolin (also known as salbutamol), the most commonly prescribed drug for asthma, works by:

1. directly widening the bronchial tree (bronchodilation)
2. stimulating respiratory drive
3. killing bacteria
4. DNA mutagenesis

Answer: 1. Ventolin is a God-send to asthma sufferers as it can quickly abort many attacks of wheezing. It is administered in the form of a puffer which, for those of you who haven't seen one, basically looks like an over-sized breath spray container.

One of the reasons I love to treat asthma is that hugely effective treatment does not generally require pills. If you take a pill it goes into the stomach, then into the small intestine where it gets absorbed across the lining of the bowel into the blood. Once in the blood stream it penetrates into most all body tissues, often including the brain. It is therefore not surprising that a pill being taken, for instance, for a heart problem (a typical example being a drug called Inderal which is a member of a group of drugs called beta blockers) may cause side effects far removed from the heart. In the example of beta blockers these commonly cause fatigue or, even more troubling for many men, impotence. Pills are not very smart. They don't know that they are supposed to go just to the diseased organ.

But that is where treating asthma is so rewarding. Much of asthma therapy is in the form of puffers (also known as "inhalers"). Puffers are much smarter than pills and have the good sense to remain in the tissue that is diseased. Accordingly, if you take a spray of Ventolin the great majority of it stays within the confines of your lungs.

Many asthmatics are chronically undertreated and hence chronically short of breath and have just come to expect that that is the way things are, pure and simple. Which is very unfortunate because it really need not be the case.

So why would patients be undertreated? There are two main reasons. One is that patients frequently don't take the prescribed treatment. Another is that some (there's that old qualifier "some" again) doctors may not be familiar with the best treatment available. This is especially so when it comes to treating asthma. It is now very well recognized that asthmatics have underlying inflammation of the bronchial tree. Suppressing that inflammation with certain anti-inflammatory, steroid puffers such as beclomethasone (also known as Beclovent or, in its more potent form, Becloforte) substantially reduces the frequency of asthma attacks. Nonetheless, time after time I will see patients who are still being treated only when their asthma flares, never having been instructed about preventive therapy simply because their doctors were not conversant with how crucial this aspect of therapy is.

Educating doctors is a major struggle for the medical profession. Traditionally there has been no formal process for this and perhaps as a result, there are those among us, I am both embarrassed and chagrined to admit, who still practice with the same knowledge base that they had five or ten years ago. And their patients are the ones to suffer. Yet these same patients very often will have no inkling that the treatment they are getting is substandard. And why should they? How many lay people know the state of the art treatment for any given illness? Do I question everything my lawyer says about what the laws of the land are? Of course not. There has to be some trust. Lots in fact. Unfortunately, sometimes that trust is misplaced and we don't even know it.

If ever tact was in order it assuredly is when I see a patient who has clearly been significantly undertreated (never mind the occasions where they have actually been mistreated). I obviously want to make sure they get onto the right therapy, but at the same time I do not want to sound critical of their usual physician....

"Mr. Simms, I think we can improve your asthma by adjusting your therapy a bit. I'd like you to start taking a puffer called Beclovent. I think you'll notice a big improvement."

"Oh, that's great. Is this a new drug?"

"Ah, not quite. Anyhow, here's the prescription."

"But doctor, why wouldn't my family doctor have given this to me already?"

"Well," I begin, choosing my words very carefully, "perhaps your condition has worsened since your doctor last saw you so."

"No, it hasn't. It's been bad for ages."

Hmm. Better try a different approach here. "Maybe it just hasn't come up during your recent visits to him."

"But doctor, I'm always asking him what to do about my asthma."

If I beat around the bush any more he's going to leave here thinking "those doctors are always protecting each other." I don't want people to think that. Even if it is true. But what if I say something that comes back to haunt me. Maybe I'll be too direct and he'll tell his doctor that I said he screwed up. That will sure land me in hot water.

"Well, it's hard to know why you weren't put on it, but in any event let's get you started and see how you fare. If you have any questions about your previous treatment it's best if you ask your family doctor. I can only account for what I do. Your family doctor can explain why he does or does not do something. Okay?"

"Okay. Thanks. We'll see you."

Sure hope that came out alright. Can't always worry about these things. Anyhow, I've been using this approach for years now. Far as I know there hasn't been any major fallout.

And so it goes.

The combined knowledge that asthma is associated with underlying airway inflammation and that puffers are safer to use than pills has led to standard, prophylactic (preventive) therapy with an anti-inflammatory steroid puffer known as:

1. Tilade
2. Intal
3. Beclovent
4. Atrovent

Answer: 3. Hope you didn't get this wrong (if you did then look back a few paragraphs). Beclovent is a wonderful drug for treating asthma. It has the benefits of steroid pills like prednisone but without the risks. Unlike prednisone, Beclovent stays within the confines of the lung so you can hit the disease where the disease is located and not elsewhere. I should add that there are other equally good steroid puffers on the market and they go by a variety of different trade names (Pulmicort for example).

Asthmatics who have a strong allergic trigger to their attacks are often treated with:

1. Intal

2. Aspirin
3. Tagamet
4. Gravol

Answer: 1. This drug is an anti-histamine in much the same way that drugs such as Benadryl or Gravol are, but unlike those pills this is a puffer. Like the ever-so-clever Beclovent, Intal has the good sense to stay in the lungs and not go wandering elsewhere.

Chronic bronchitis and emphysema (collectively known as COPD from chronic *obstructive pulmonary disease*) are also very common causes of shortness of breath.

Typical features of COPD include all of the following except:

1. a long history of smoking
2. a barrel-shaped chest
3. frequent wheezing
4. alpha-1-antitrypsin deficiency

Answer: 4. This metabolic defect can indeed cause COPD (and should be tested for in any "COPDer" who has never been a smoker), but it is a very rare, not typical, finding.

What both asthma and COPD (which used to be called COLD-chronic *obstructive lung disease* — thankfully the moniker has changed! Used to drive me crazy when I would get a call from the emerg to see a patient said to have "a cold") have in common is narrowing of the airways (that is, the bronchial tree) but in asthma this tends to be reversible whereas in COPD it tends to be fixed.

The great majority of patients with COPD have been chronic smokers. And many of these patients, even with well-established lung disease and even though feeling short of breath with only minimal exertion, still puff away. "I just can't quit," they tell me. Now if ever I deserved an Oscar nomination it is surely when I have to deal with this. I try ever so hard to follow the rules. *Don't be judgmental. Don't be professorial. Don't be antagonistic. Do be compassionate. Do be understanding.* Sort of like medical "Romper Room."

So, like a good little doctor, I turn on my encouragement mode and say, "Have you thought about quitting? Oh, good. Have you actually stopped at all? A couple of weeks, huh. Last year. Well, that's great. You proved you could do it. Now you just have to try again. I'm sure you know lots of people who tried and failed before they eventually got off cigarettes altogether." I listen for silent applause. Thank you, thank you.

Well, it may be acting, but results matter and the truth is, it works. It really does work. A non-judgmental, encouraging approach does truly help in getting patients to quit smoking.

But inside I'm doing a slow burn. *You shmuck. Here I am doing my best to keep you healthy and you go out and wreck it by puffing away. Why do I bother?* But I do bother. And you know why? Because when one of my patients who smokes succeeds in quitting I get so excited I could cry. True story. I can feel my tears welling up. Suck, eh? Oh well. I look at this patient in front of me and I know that my encouragement and yes, my acting skill, has effected a change that could do more for them than any drug I could possibly prescribe. As my eight-year-old would say, "YES!!"

Oh, one other thing about smoking that I've learned over the years. Never confine questioning about smoking to just "do you smoke?" Patient after patient will answer in the negative. Which will mislead you if you don't follow up that question with "have you ever smoked?" at which point I will then commonly find out that the patient had indeed stopped smoking — about four hours earlier.

Asking patients about their alcohol consumption is another very tricky thing. Naive sole that I was, I used to approach it very straightforwardly.

"Do you drink?" I would ask. If answered in the affirmative (a truism: patients who say they never drink, never do. Patients who say they drink "just a little" may or may not drink just a little) I would then ask how much they drank and draw up an estimate of the number of drinks consumed per day. Trouble was, such estimates were grossly inaccurate and patients typically reacted defensively when approached in this manner. So as time went by I learned about newer and better strategies.

Firstly, it is best to ask about alcohol consumption immediately after having asked about the patient's smoking history. People accept questions about smoking as being part and parcel of a medical history. If these questions are then followed by queries regarding alcohol patients rightly assume that the two go together; that is, the doctor is doing a general inquiry with regard to lifestyle factors that can impact on one's health. And that way, people are less likely to feel that the doctor is asking them about alcohol because the physician suspects they are alcoholics. Even if they do.

Secondly, is use of something called the CAGE questionnaire. You may well recognize its component parts if you've ever talked to your doctor about drinking. The patient is asked if they have ever felt that they should Cut down on what they drink. And if they have ever been Annoyed by people commenting on their drinking. (N.B. Not if *they* have annoyed other people.) And if they ever feel Guilty about drinking. And lastly, if they ever have an Eye opener in the morning to get going. A score of two or more gives a more than 75 percent likelihood of the patient being an alcoholic. If the CAGE questionnaire is asked in a non-judgmental manner patients almost without exception respond accurately.

On occasion I will see a patient who vehemently denies having a problem with alcohol despite a high score on the questionnaire. This inconsistency is particularly striking when I find out that they are taking Antabuse. (Antabuse is a drug sometimes used to treat alcoholism. If you take Antabuse and then consume alcohol, you will, to put it indelicately but honestly, puke your guts out.) Denial, denial, denial.

Looking after patients with alcohol-related diseases tests the mettle of even the most resilient physician. I know that alcoholism is a disease. I know that it is an addiction. I know all of that and other doctors know all of that. But can you imagine the frustration of treating someone for their cirrhosis of the liver or their internal bleeding or their leg edema or one of a myriad of other alcohol-related problems only to have them then go out and do their best to undo all that you've just done your best to correct? Sometimes I think life would be easier if I could delude myself into looking at such self-destructive patients as being like automobiles driven by reckless drivers; the auto body shop probably doesn't complain that they've got a steady customer, so why should a physician? But we do. Drives us crazy in fact. Guess we're not as mercenary as the press sometimes makes us out to be. Sort of reminds me of a summer job a friend of mine had when he was a teenager. He spent the entire month of July moving the contents of a warehouse from one part of the building to another. And spent the entire month of August putting things back where they started after the manager had changed his mind. My friend got paid regardless. But no job satisfaction there. Just frustration.

Irene Brett was a fifty-five-year-old long-standing diabetic. Recently she had noticed that when walking through the local mall she would start to feel short of breath. It would quickly clear once she had rested for a few minutes only to start up again as soon as she resumed walking. She had gone to her family doctor and had had a chest x-ray, some blood work and pulmonary function tests (wherein one blows into a machine that can record and graph the depth and velocity of a breath). Nothing abnormal was found. She was reassured that nothing seemed seriously amiss, however her breathing progressively worsened and she was therefore sent to see me.

On the subject of referrals to consultants (and just before we get back to Mrs. Brett), have you ever wondered, if you need specialty care, how your doctor decides which consultant to refer you to? The best one around of course. Well, sometimes. If the truth be told, the consultant's ability is only one factor and frequently not a key one. Often more important is whether the consultant and the family doctor are friends. Or if the family doctor knows that he'll never get his urgent cases seen promptly if he does not send the specialist elective patients. Or if the consultant is renting office space from the family doctor and for obvious reasons there is strong motivation to keep the specialist busy.

A number of years ago there was a doctors' strike in Ontario. Some physicians thought the strike was ill-advised and counter-productive. And said so. I remember speaking with one such physician, a general surgeon in a fairly small town. After voicing his opinion to his colleagues, he quickly found his referrals to taper off; so much so that he debated moving to another community. Things did eventually turn around for him, but it took almost five years before the blackballing totally abated. What amazed him the most was how so many physicians who had felt that he could look after their patients quite competently one day suddenly felt that he could not the next. Like, why else would they possibly have stopped sending him patients?

So now, back to Mrs. Brett.

She appeared to be in generally good health apart from her diabetes. She denied (funny expression that doctors use — sounds like the patient is on the witness stand; perhaps in a way they are) any other symptoms and her examination (another peculiar expression — it is, of course, not the patient's examination, but the doctor's examination of the patient) was normal.

The next step should be to:

1. do an exercise stress test
2. reassure Mrs. Brett that she is healthy and could safely forego further tests
3. repeat the chest x-ray (to make sure no interval change had occurred)
4. send her for psychiatric assessment for a probable anxiety disorder

Answer: 1. An exercise stress test involves walking on a gradually quickening (and inclining) treadmill whilst electrocardiograms (EKGs) are performed. Since breathlessness can be due to cardiac disease and since Mrs. Brett's lungs were okay, her heart had to be checked out further; hence the need for the stress test.

At three minutes into the test she complained of increasing shortness of breath (also known as SOB. Acronyms and medicine seem to go hand in hand. My favourite is "LOL in NAD with

SOB" referring to a little old lady in no acute distress with shortness of breath).

Just as Mrs. Brett told me she was having a hard time breathing I started to feel the same way. For I was looking at her EKG and it showed profound and worrisome abnormalities. We stopped the treadmill and within a few minutes we both felt well again. It was now clear that she had heart disease and in particular, disease of the coronary arteries, but rather than manifesting as chest pain, it was giving her breathlessness.

Some people with coronary artery disease don't get any symptoms at all. This is termed:

1. electrocardiographic instability
2. coronary vasculitis
3. pectus excavatum
4. silent angina

Answer: 4. It is of course an oxymoron (the classic, if over-used example of an oxymoron being the term "military intelligence") to say angina is silent, but let's not get too picky.

During exercise the heart has to work harder. And like any machine, if it is doing more work it needs more fuel. But if you have coronary artery disease then the arteries to your heart are clogged with cholesterol and so the flow of blood (the fuel) can't increase to keep up with the demands of your exercising heart (the machine). In most people this mismatch leads to chest pain (angina). There are, however, patients such as Mrs. Brett in whom typical angina does not occur. Moreover, if portable EKG studies (Holter monitoring) are done on patients with known coronary artery disease, many of these patients, whether they have diabetes or not, will show evidence of anginal episodes which were totally symptom-free. The difficulty for the physician is knowing how to gauge response to treatment if someone's problem is not associated with symptoms. Keep someone hooked up to a heart monitor for the rest of their lives? Might make me feel better, but I have a feeling that my patients might object.

Chapter Thirteen

Sore Throats, Second Opinions, and Fragile Egos

One of the most common symptoms leading to a visit to a family doctor is sore throat. Although sore throats are usually pretty straightforward, like much else in medicine things are sometimes more complicated than they appear at first.

"Strep throat" is a throat infection that most people have had at one time or another.

Strep throat is caused by:

1. a virus
2. a bacteria
3. a fungus
4. all of the above

Answer: 2.

The full name for the germ causing strep throat is:

1. streptococcus viridans

2. streptococcus bovis
3. group A, beta hemoltyic streptococcus
4. untypable streptococcus

Answer: 3.

Complications due to strep throat include all of the following *except*:

1. rheumatoid arthritis
2. rheumatic fever
3. Quinsy (an abscess behind the tonsil)
4. kidney failure

Answer: 1.

Remarkably few people (including physicians) realize that treating a strep throat with penicillin does not hasten recovery from the sore throat itself; the pain goes away just as fast without antibiotics. (How come doctors don't know this simple fact? How come I didn't know it myself until about two months ago? Wellll, no one ever told me. And I had never seen an article mentioning it. Poor excuses? Certainly. But you can't know everything; even every simple thing. Hence yet another reason why doctors tend not to criticize one another.) Antibiotics are used, therefore, not to lessen symptoms, but rather, to decrease the likelihood of complications developing.

In order to definitively diagnose if pharyngitis (throat inflammation) is bacterial one must do which of the following?

1. a throat swab
2. a blood count
3. a chest x-ray
4. a full physical examination

Answer: 1. A throat swab is the only reliable way to establish if pharyngitis is bacterial in origin.

John was an eighteen-year-old high school student. He had presented to his family doctor with a sore, red throat. A throat swab was taken and, pending the result, he was started on penicillin. The next day the swab was reported as being negative (that is, sterile) and the antibiotic was discontinued. After a few days John felt no better and indeed felt somewhat worse so he returned to the doctor's office. He complained of having had fevers and sweats and upon examination his doctor noticed that John not only had swollen lymph glands in his neck, but also in his armpits (the "axillae") and groins.

These new findings would suggest that John had:

1. a resistant strep which required a different antibiotic
2. mono ("infectious mononucleosis")
3. leukemia
4. diphtheria

Answer: 2.

When we think about mono we generally think about fevers, sweats, malaise, fatigue, and swelling of the lymph glands. What we often do not think about is that mono can cause one of the worst sore throats imaginable. Beefy red, lots of pus, and, in rare cases, tonsils so big they result in a positive Bell Canada sign: reaching out and touching one another. But in this case reaching out isn't an act of love, but rather is an act of inflammation. Inflammation so severe that the tonsils can totally obstruct the airway potentially leading to asphyxiation. Some affected individuals need to have a tracheotomy to allow air to get down into the lungs. Fortunately, even though antibiotics are to no avail in treating mono, the inflammation in the throat can respond amazingly to, what else, anti-inflammatory medication. But not the small potatoes. Rather, the big guns — corticosteroids. In particular, drugs akin to prednisone. Ahhh prednisone, wonder drug of the century ... so long as it is used with the greatest respect.

Bill was a thirty-year-old man who, over the span of forty-eight hours developed an intensely sore throat. Every swallow was agonizing. He went to his family doctor who carefully inspected Bill's throat and found ... nothing. No inflammation. No swelling. No lymph gland enlargement. Nothing.

Bill was reassured and sent home but, feeling no better, he returned to the family doctor's office a few days later. His throat remained intensely sore and he had started to feel generally unwell. Figuring that Bill must have a bacterial pharyngitis even though his throat looked quite fine, Bill's family doctor started him on penicillin. (I must make an aside here. Penicillin was one of the first antibiotics around. It is decades old. There is a tendency in medicine amongst both practioners and patients to assume that what is new is good and what is old is lousy. What a shame. After several decades guess what the best drug in the world is for the treatment of strep throat? You got it. Penicillin.)

A week later Bill was still sick and he requested a second opinion. His family doctor was agreeable and soon thereafter Bill was in to see me.

By now he had been ill for almost two weeks. And that was to my advantage. For by the time I had been asked to see him he had developed the additional findings of ten-pound weight loss, tremor, diarrhea, and a very tender thyroid gland which, when taken together, allowed me to quickly arrive at a diagnosis.

Bill was suffering from:

  1. a bacterial infection of the thyroid
  2. hypothyroidism
  3. Grave's Disease
  4. subacute thyroiditis

Answer: 4. Subacute thyroiditis is a viral infection of the thyroid gland. Typically, it causes pain not only in the thyroid but radiating all the way up to the throat.

In subacute thyroiditis the thyroid gland becomes inflamed and releases thyroid hormone which is normally stored in the gland. Sort of like air escaping from a punctured balloon. As a result, people get symptoms both from the viral infection itself (fever, sweats, malaise, a tender thyroid) and from the increased thyroid hormone levels in the blood (weight loss, tremor, diarrhea).

The moral of the story is twofold:

One: the disease is not necessarily where the pain is located. (Witness the numerous heart attack patients who have pain not in the chest, but in the jaw or the arm.)

Two: it is much easier to be the consultant than to be the family doctor. The family doctor typically sees things fresh, just as the symptoms are beginning. On the other hand, the consultant generally sees the patient only after some time has elapsed; time enough to have often allowed symptoms to have evolved into a nice, clear-cut picture. In fact this is so frequently the case that it is often counter productive to see patients too quickly after they have been referred. If a patient, say with a bit of a fever, is seen by me the same day that their doctor has initiated the referral then not enough time will have passed to have allowed the great majority of self-limited febrile illnesses (such as most virus infections) to have spontaneously corrected.

When I relayed to Bill's family doctor what I had diagnosed he was thankful that things had been sorted out, but frustrated that he had not come up with the diagnosis himself, and even more frustrated that the patient had been the one to have requested the second opinion. Bad enough to feel you can't figure something out; even worse when the patient realizes you can't and is the one to initiate a second opinion. Worst of all when the person giving the second opinion readily comes up with the answer.

Second opinions can be a difficult thing for a doctor's ego. Certainly if a doctor is secure and confident and if it is the doctor initiating the second opinion on a difficult case then the whole thing is taken in stride. So that takes care of one case in a thousand. Now what about the rest? What about the doctor who is perhaps not always quite so secure and confident and when it is the patient that is the one requesting (or indeed, demanding) the second opinion on a case that is not particularly complex...?

"So, Mrs. Levesque, as we were discussing earlier, your heart rhythm disorder is nothing to worry about. Your bout of atrial fibrillation has long since passed and the tests have all come back normal. I'd recommend that you just do your best to forget about it. If your symptoms come back, well then of course let me know right away."

"But doctor, can you be completely sure that there isn't anything else going on?"

"Well, we've done all the necessary studies and nothing else has shown up. There's no evidence of coronary artery disease, your blood pressure is excellent, the thyroid checked out okay. No, I really don't think there is anything else going on here."

"You know doctor, it's not that I don't trust you, but maybe I should get another opinion. Just to be extra careful."

Adopting the most professional approach I can muster, I reply "by all means Mrs. Levesque. Don't worry, I don't take it personally." In other words, I lie.

Because I *do* take it personally. Here you have a patient saying they trust you then, in the same breath, saying something clearly indicating they do not *really* trust you. So why shouldn't it be taken personally?

The coup de grace is when the patient then asks, "Oh, and when should I come back to see you?"

"Never. If you don't trust me now I know you are always going to be questioning what I do and say in the future. I don't need that kind of aggravation. Good-bye."

Which translates into "Oh, that won't be necessary. I'll send your family doctor a letter. Should be there in a few days. If he feels you need to come back I'd be pleased to see you again."

Intellectually I can certainly understand why patients might want a second opinion. People know that doctors are fallible. Very fallible. So why wouldn't they want another opinion? Maybe it's surprising that they don't all want another opinion. I do wonder, though, how crucial that second opinion would be if they had to pay for it.

The other fascinating thing about "the second opinion" is how unerring it is. Which is fine with me when I'm the one giving the second opinion, but not quite so fine otherwise. Without exception, the doctor offering the second opinion is thought by the patient to have given the definitive conclusion. If it differs from the first opinion, well, I guess the first doctor just got it wrong. Funny thing, this.

Chapter Fourteen

HIGH BLOOD PRESSURE, HIGH OVERHEAD, AND HIGHLY IMPORTANT ASSORTED MISCELLANEA

"My blood pressure is up."

"How do you know?"

"My face is flushed and I've got a headache. And I feel really nervous and shaky."

"I see."

"It must be very high," Debbie said, looking at me expectantly.

"Well Debbie, your blood pressure might be up. Or it might not be. Lets check."

I took the blood pressure cuff off the wall and wrapped it around Debbie's arm. As I rapidly inflated then slowly deflated the cuff, I realized Debbie was eyeing me intently.

"Its one-twenty over eighty," I said.

"Is that good?" Debbie asked.

"Yes, its perfectly normal."

"But what about my symptoms?"

"I guess we'll have to look elsewhere for a cause. They're not due to high blood pressure."

Was I right?

    1. yes (clue: remember who authored this book)
    2. no

Answer: 1. What else did you expect.

Debbie's blood pressure was 120/80. If it had been higher, say 150/90, might that have explained her symptoms?

    1. yes
    2. no

Answer: 2. High blood pressure almost never causes symptoms. When it does, it is only if the readings are sky high (like 240/140) or, if it is somewhat less severe (say, 180/110), but has come on very rapidly.

Hypertension is usually caused by:

    1. stress
    2. obesity
    3. smoking
    4. unknown factors

Answer: 4. Ninety-five percent of the time we do not know the cause of high blood pressure. We do know that certain things can *aggravate* high blood pressure such as stress, obesity, sedentariness, caffeine, salt, alcohol, and smoking, but these factors in and of themselves do not *cause* it.

Ever wonder exactly what a normal blood pressure reading is? Keep wondering. There is no such thing as an universally accepted "normal" reading. Rather, there is a fairly wide range of *acceptable* readings all the way up to 140 (or so) systolic, 90 (or so) diastolic. I specifically indicate "or so" because what is considered acceptable keeps changing. When I started medical school I was taught that acceptable was up to 160 systolic, 95 diastolic. When I was a resident I was taught that acceptable was up to 150 systolic, 90 diastolic. Now, in the 1990s we are told that acceptable is up to 140 systolic, 90 diastolic. And in the next century...?

Is there such a thing as abnormally low blood pressure? Well if you are deathly ill with shock (true shock such as with hemorrhaging or a severe heart attack, not just being "upset") certainly one has abnormally low blood pressure. But in someone who is not acutely ill, low blood pressure is not a disease. Absolutely not. At least absolutely not in North America. In Germany low blood pressure is considered a frequent cause of symptoms such as lassitude and fatigue and indeed is one of the most commonly treated ailments. Both North American and German physicians have access to the same medical literature. Same information. Different diagnoses and treatment. And such is the state of the art of medicine.

As I mentioned in an earlier chapter doctors are often justifiably criticized for not taking the time to fully (or sometimes even partially) explain things. For example, people will commonly be told simply that their blood pressure is "okay" or "just a bit up" or "not in a worrisome range" without any further elaboration. Which is probably quite adequate for some people, but certainly not for the majority. What exactly does "a bit up" or "not worrisome" really mean? It should most definitely not be construed as meaning harmless because even a "bit" of high blood pressure can be hazardous in the long run.

Let's say that you have no history of hypertension, but when you go for your annual check-up your doctor finds your blood pressure to be elevated at 170/90.

The next step should be to:

1. start blood pressure pills
2. start lifestyle change (exercising, weight loss, etc)
3. come back in a few weeks
4. come back in a year

Answer: 3. High blood pressure on a single occasion does *not* establish a diagnosis. Many people do not realize that blood pressure is dynamic, not static. And because it is a constantly changing entity, it should be checked at least three times over the span of a few weeks or months before you are labelled as "having" high blood pressure. Labels are hard to shake; especially once your life insurance company hears about them.

Your doctor asks you to come back a few times over the next two months to see if your blood pressure is persistingly elevated. Unfortunately, it is. You are, however, an inherently sceptical person and you wonder if the doctor's measurements are truly accurate. Having a company nurse where you work, you decide to have her check your pressure a few times. Lo and behold, she finds your blood pressure to be completely normal.

Why might this discrepancy be present?

1. you have "white coat hypertension"
2. the nurse and the doctor have different size blood pressure cuffs

3. the doctor has better hearing than the nurse
4. all of the above

Answer: 4. There are many technical factors influencing blood pressure measurements. For example, doctors typically get higher readings than do nurses because patients generally feel more stressed when seeing physicians (so called "white coat hypertension"). Also, if your arm is particularly big or small then the conventionally sized blood pressure cuffs will give false readings. And hearing the ("Koratkoff") sounds with the stethoscope depends of course on having a reasonable stethoscope and hearing.

So now you are really confused. Do you or do you not have high blood pressure?

"Whose readings are the reliable ones; the doctor's or the nurse's?" you wonder. The accurate readings are likely the:

1. nurse's
2. doctor's
3. both

Answer: 3. Truth of the matter is they are likely both accurate. Accurate in the sense of indicating what your blood pressure is at that moment in time.

So then, how will it be decided if you have high blood pressure or not?

Well, that can be very tricky. To just pass off the doctor's readings as being aberrant because you were under stress when you were there would be to ignore the simple fact that quite possibly the stress that you experience when seeing the doctor may not be too dissimilar to much of the stress you experience a substantial portion of your waking hours. Maybe your pressure is up a fair bit of the time. On the other hand, maybe it is not.

There are a number of ways you can sort out this all too common conundrum:

Strategy A: Wear a portable blood pressure cuff for twenty-four hours. Such a cuff automatically inflates (and deflates of course) every hour of the day and night and thus gives an impression of how things are around the clock. Not recommended if you are giving an important presentation the following day.

Strategy B: Buy your own blood pressure cuff and keep an eye on your own readings. Not recommended for the obsessive-compulsive.

Strategy C: Just rely on your doctor's readings. Oh what a trusting soul you are.

Strategy D: Just rely on your workplace nurse's readings. Ditto.

Strategy E: Undergo a careful search for evidence of hypertension having damaged your body (for examples; having tests to look for heart enlargement or kidney damage)

Strategy F: Say "to hell with all this" and ignore the problem. A remarkably common approach. (But not recommended).

In practice, it is often some combination of these strategies that ends up being used with the particular approach being tailored to the individual patient. For example, if I have someone with consistently high office readings, but normal values at home, it becomes clear that they do indeed have hypertension if there is evidence of heart enlargement on an electrocardiogram or cardiac ultrasound. Conversely, if someone seems otherwise perfectly healthy and if a twenty-four-hour blood pressure study is normal I will take my office readings with a grain of salt (which I can safely do since my blood pressure is normal; or at least it was when I last had it checked several years ago. Typical doctor, eh? Routine check-ups. Nah, they're for other people).

It's actually quite amazing how often health care professionals use the wrong size cuff when measuring someone's blood pressure. Sometimes this is because the doctor (or nurse) doesn't realize that if the blood pressure cuff is the wrong size it will give inaccurate results. And sometimes the doctor is just too cheap to buy a variety of blood pressure cuffs.

Doctors cheap? Well, I hate to make generalizations (actually I don't hate to make generalizations, it's just that they get you in trouble so darn quickly), but some (there's that word again) doctors *are* cheap. Amazing, that. Doctors earn a good living. A very good living. So why do so many doctors have the cheapest furniture and office equipment around? Well, there is a simple explanation for that. Fancier furnishings do not generate fancier revenue. Not very many patients are likely to change doctors because they don't like the office decor.

Speaking about office decor, have you ever wondered why it is that waiting room magazines are so hopelessly outdated? It's usually because the people working in the doctor's office (including the doctor) rarely go into the waiting room and more specifically, never pick up the magazines themselves. So it's not part of their consciousness. It never occurs to them. Or if it does, what incentive is there to change the status quo? Are patients not going to come back if the magazines are not current?

The other day, after all my patients had left, I sat down in my own waiting room. Just sat there. *Hmm, the music is kind of loud. Stain on that chair — doesn't look very professional. Advertising brochures for a contractor — how did those get in here? Lighting's too dark — no wonder why people are falling asleep out here.* I felt like I was a voyeur. Seeing things from a perspective I had never had before. Oh, by the way, if you're in need of any 1985 issues of *Time* magazine, I have lots for you to choose from.

And what of the secretary in a doctor's office? From the physician's perspective a secretary who gets all the work done promptly and efficiently is a God-send. Truth of the matter is, the secretary's interaction with patients is often less important. Not unimportant, just less important. Patients may love or hate the secretary, but it is rare indeed that a patient will not return even if you have the rudest of secretaries.

Which is not to say that a secretary's demeanour cannot affect the doctor's practice and in particular, practice volume. One of my specialist colleagues, after hiring a new secretary, noticed his waiting list to be growing shorter and shorter. He griped to me about it and I happened to mention it to my own secretary.

"No surprise to me," she said.

"Really? Why is that?" I asked.

"Have you ever spoken to her?"

"Yes, I guess I did once."

"And. What did you think?"

"Sounded pleasant enough to me," I answered.

"Sure does," Carol answered. "But when she talks to one of us; you know, one of us lowly secretaries, she's a rude bitch. There's no way I'm going to send our patients to see Dr. Pearson if it means having to book an appointment with that secretary of his. And the rest of the secretaries feel the same way I do."

Well, someone must have told Dr. Pearson what had been happening because he eventually fired her. Which must have been very tough on both of them. In fact, I think shortly after that they got divorced.

Before I went into practice I had been under the impression that the dynamics of what took place in a doctor's office were fairly well confined to what went on between the patient and the doctor in the privacy of the examining room. To paraphrase the late Jackie Gleason, "how wrong I was!" Indeed, there were a number of nuances I would quickly learn. Nuances that, at times, resemble well, choreographed dance steps. Some examples:

The Ventriloquist: The secretary calls the patient to the window and asks
for the biographic information, at which point the ventriloquist, a
relative who accompanied the patient, answers the questions.
Performed by males and females alike. Generally speaking, this
dance has been perfected long before the visit to the doctor with
many years of practice having been garnered at social gatherings.

The Nospeaketenglish: The relative explains that the patient does not
speak English and thus needs the relative to interpret. The doctor
asks the patient if she is having any symptoms. The patient starts to
answer in quite adequate English, but is interrupted by the relative
who then tells the physician that they will interpret at which point
the relative then turns to the patient and says, in English but with
foreign inflection, the same question the doctor had asked. Ver
batim. The relative is then asked by the doctor, politely but firmly,
to leave. The relative gets upset. The patient gets upset. The doctor
gets upset. The relative stays. The interview takes twice as long as it
would have without the help of the relative. The doctor sulks.

The Same Name Two-Step: The doctor calls the patient in from the
waiting room and is then greeted by two people who, incredible as
this may seem, have the same name. Especially astounding is the
fact that often they are of differing sexes yet may both go by a quite
gender-specific name such as Mary or John. This dance tends to be
performed simultaneously with The Ventriloquist and in fact
judges often have a hard time distinguishing which performance
they are watching.

The Mommy Dearest: A particularly popular dance, The Mommy Dearest
is show-cased by the adult female of the homo-sapien species who
brings, without having requested consent from the physician, her
maternal progenitor into the examining room during the initial visit
to the doctor. As the interview with the patient is necessarily
detailed and, as the physician is generally of the nature that history
taking should not be hindered by the presence of patient-selected
spectators, The Mommy Dearest often engenders some discomfort
among its practitioners as they dance to questions about sexual
activity, vaginal discharge, and the like.

The Idunnohedidnsay: Well recognized by medical practitioners
throughout history, this classic dance is performed by people of all
ages so long as they are able to inflect the tail end of their sentences
with an upward lilt. Typically a two-part step with the initial move
by the physician telling the patient at the conclusion of the exam

that the patient is to book a return appointment with the receptionist for, as an example, two weeks later. The second step is performed immediately after the first with the patient, upon being asked by the receptionist when the next visit is to be, responding in a carefully modulated voice, that "Idunnohedidnsay."

Not infrequently, people will complain about having had to wait several weeks to get an appointment to see a specialist. To hear such a complaint is quite frustrating. Do people think that doctors derive pleasure from making people defer getting seen? I did, however, find a great way to deflect such criticism. In the truest sense of, ahem, spin doctoring, when patients disparagingly comment that "you sure are busy doctor, it took three weeks to get in to see you," I simply reply "yes, you're right. But would you want to see a doctor that wasn't busy?" Works like a charm.

Speaking about waiting, have you ever wondered why it is that you wait (and wait and wait and ...) in a doctor's office? Although there can be a multitude of reasons some factors are much more common than others:

Tales of the Unexpected: Before most patients walk into the office the doctor rarely knows if the person is there for a minor complaint or for something which initially seems to be minor but in fact turns out to be much more serious (and time consuming) than expected. As such, patients are typically booked at fixed intervals and when the unexpected happens, that delays everything. "Why," you might ask, "would the doctor not just book more time with each patient so that if the unexpected happens, there will be time to deal with it?" Good question. Glad you asked. The answer is twofold: Firstly, to book extra time between each patient would cause the physician to spend a lot of time twiddling his or her thumbs (and boredom doesn't pay well under the fee schedule). Secondly, it would increase the length of time to get an appointment to see the doctor in the first place. I should also add that obstetricians always have the perfect alibi; I mean, who could possibly deny their right to be late to the office because they were in the process of catching a baby? The fact that perhaps what they were actually catching was some gossip in the doctors' lounge; well, who's going to know, eh?

Disorganized? Who, Me?: Some doctors have all the smarts in the world, but are terribly disorganized. They lose track of the time when they are seeing patients or when they get called to the phone. Some such individuals cope only because they have that most important of assets, an organized secretary. Often however, organized secretaries quit these offices out of sheer frustration.

Looking Out for Number One: My father-in-law, a very meticulous individual, has never been late for an appointment in his life. And he expects to be treated likewise. So it drove him around the bend when he was referred to a specialist, got there at eight in the morning (he was scheduled for the first slot of the day) and walked into a waiting room full of patients booked for the same time. It wasn't a scheduling error. No, the doctor was of the mind that in case someone didn't show (and no patient, no money) best to have ample back-up. More than ample in fact. It didn't even occur to him that other people considered their time as valuable as his was.

My Mother Taught Me to be Polite: My wife is a physician. Although she works the same number of hours per day as most doctors, she sees about half the number of patients. That way she can spend twice as much time with each one. She listens to their complaints patiently. She listens. And listens. And listens. She knows that they have a story to tell and she lets them tell it. She does not believe in rushing her patients. So despite booking longer appointments with patients than most any other doctor would dream of doing, she still ends up running late (often, very late). Her patients love her for her patience and rarely complain about waiting to see her because they know that once they are in her office, they too will be able to say their piece, have all their questions answered and will come away feeling satisfied with the attention and care they have received. Having three kids, a mortgage, and a car loan, it is a very good thing that my wife is married to a doctor.

The Combo Platter: Most patients wait. Most doctors keep them waiting. And assuredly most doctors do not pigeon-hole neatly into one of the categories above. Rather, it is often one reason one moment and another some other time. Some days we are disorganized. Some days we're stuck at the hospital with a sick patient. Some days the computer crashes and we know that, gee well, if we try this or maybe that, you know, it's going to be back running in a second and I'll get right to that next patient. And some days, like today, you've just *got* to finish one more paragraph of that book you've been working on.

Occasionally a patient will get so fed up with repeated marathon sessions in a chronically tardy doctor's office that they change physicians. Other times a patient may switch for purely pragmatic reasons such as how close the office is to the house or workplace, if the office hours are convenient, if a prompt appointment is given when you're feeling ill, and so on. Some people leave a doctor because they find him or her to have a disagreeable personality. And sometimes there are factors like that noticed by a physician friend of mine who observed that 10 percent of his patients entered his practice because he was Jewish and 10 percent of his patients left his practice because he was Jewish (no, not the same 10 percent).

You may have noticed that absent from this list of reasons for changing doctors is anything to do with the quality of care the doctor is providing. I am amazed (though I know I should not be) by the number of people I see that go to doctors who are, to put it kindly, not likely to be receiving the Nobel Prize for Medicine and Physiology. But they have busy practices and their patients love them. Why? Because the doctor is nice. Very nice. Well, I'll tell you something. Nice is nice, but if I'm sick I'd rather go to the biggest son of a bitch in the world if he is more likely to figure out what's wrong with me and get me better. Problem is, how is the average person to know that the one doctor is more skilled than the other?

Wise people will try to choose their physician based on at least some basic investigative work. And well they should. At the very least you should canvass friends, neighbours, or relatives for recommendations. If you know a nurse who works at the nearby hospital she will likely have a sense of which physicians are on the ball. Whatever you do, **do not** just pick out names from the yellow pages. Lots of people do just that.

If you have lots of *chutzpah* (the quintessential example of *chutzpah* being the son who kills his parents and then pleads for clemency now that he is an orphan) you could try the following technique. When next in need of medical attention go to the emergency department (don't tell them I sent you) and, when the emerg doc is examining you let him (or her) know that you are looking for a family doctor and, if he (or she of course) has no objection, would he (or she of course) tell you who his (or her — gee this is getting to be a nuisance) doctor is. They may tell you or they may not. If you're lucky they will. There's no guarantee that their family doctor is excellent, but you've certainly improved your odds. Dollars to donuts the physician that other physicians seek out is not a medical neanderthal.

Sometimes I am tempted to tell a patient that they really would be better served by changing physicians. If you promise not to tell any of my referring physicians I'll even let you in on a deep, dark secret. I once actually did recommend to someone that they change doctors. And you know what? They looked at me as if I was crazy. They loved their doctor. Change to someone else? Why didn't I mind my own business anyhow? O-o-o-kay. Won't try that again.

In the same way that it disturbs me to see patients blindly trusting certain doctors, it also disturbs me to see patients who clearly do not recognize that their physician is excellent. There is an emergency room physician ("casualty officer") I know who is unbelievably skilled. When he refers a patient to you it is never a "slough," never inappropriate, never less than fully worked-up. Indeed, Dr. Henry Davis is brilliant at quickly and efficiently sorting out and treating even the toughest of emergency cases. Not to overdo this, but I really mean it when I say that every other physician in town (including his fellow casualty officers) would hope that it was Dr. Davis's shift if we had the misfortune of becoming acutely ill. Okay. I think I've painted the picture for you. And I know you're now waiting for the other shoe to drop.

Well, here's the other shoe. This doctor is not a man of many words; indeed he tends to be curt with patients. And can be arrogant. And he dresses like a slob. And often does not explain things as fully as he should. He is certainly not intentionally rude, but as he once told me, he "doesn't like to play the game." He sees his role as being to figure out what is wrong with someone and get them better as quickly and efficiently as possible. He does not see his role as trying to resemble Marcus Welby. He cares deeply about the patients he looks after but showing it is another thing.

It's really no surprise that this refusing to role-play has landed him, more than once, in hot water. Patients will commonly, after he leaves their room, turn to the nurse and say "who the hell was that guy?" And the nurse will then have to explain that "that guy" was an excellent emergency room physician, the best around. However, patients often don't see it that way. For them, he was just a rude shmuck. And all the explaining in the world isn't likely to change that impression. Shame really. But I don't blame patients for seeing it that way. How in the world are they to know that he has made a clever diagnosis, or interpreted a difficult EKG, or given them the best treatment?

I think if there is a moral to this story it is simply this. Being the best doctor in the world means one thing to that small group of people who are able to judge your academic abilities. And means something profoundly different to that immensely larger community who must make their judgments based on your persona; do you listen? are you friendly? do you not only care but appear to care? and so forth. That may be the moral here, but it certainly is not very satisfying. Not to down-play the importance of these traits in a physician. No one could possibly disagree that a "nice" doctor is *nice* to have, but the truth of the matter is that the skills behind the exterior trappings are a heck of a lot more important when you're lying on a stretcher with a heart attack.

Some people think that it is a great idea to be friends with your doctor. Not necessarily bosom buddies, but friends nonetheless. I notice this particularly with men similar in age to myself. They'll call me by my first name. And talk to me as if they are not really in the office because they are ill; no they are actually there just to shoot the breeze. Which wouldn't bother me at all except that the closer my personal relationship is with a patient the lesser is my ability to properly care for them; yet they don't realize this.

This hit home when a neighbourhood friend of mine suddenly developed internal bleeding. His wife called me over to his house and I went with him to the hospital. I remember trying to resuscitate him in the emergency department and feeling like I was flailing about. I couldn't get the I.V. started. I couldn't pass the stomach tube. A poor performance if ever I saw one. Thankfully, one of the surgeons happened by, quickly figured out what was going on and relieved me of my duties.

After the dust had settled, the surgeon took me aside and said, "Look Ian, you were too close to him. You can't look after a friend. At least not competently." I sat down and realized that he was absolutely right. The take-home message: if you become friends with your doctor do both of you a favour and change doctors.

If it serves no one well to have friends as patients, then it is even worse to have relatives as patients. Fortunately most doctors and their relatives recognize this. What does happen, however, is that physicians get called upon to act as an intermediary between their relatives and their relatives' doctors.

A few years ago my grandfather became very ill. He was admitted to hospital and deteriorated to the point that he needed to be put on a life support system. Throughout this time my relatives relied on me to communicate with the attending physician to discuss my grandfather's status. Which I did. And so I was told about his pneumonia and his confusion, his worsening kidney function and his stroke; the list went on and on. With precise detail the myriad of maladies besetting him were recounted to me. And it was up to me to then convert the medicalese to lay language for the rest of the family's benefit. Which I did. And when it came time to decide about withdrawing the ventilator, it was up to me to discuss this with the ICU staff. Which I did.

And during that whole process; the initial illness and the subsequent worsening, the admission to ICU and the downward spiral leading to death, my family grieved. But I did not. They cried. But I did not.

It was not until my grandfather's funeral that I wept. I wept for him and for my loss. But I also wept because I had been cheated. For weeks my family had been mourning, but I had not been allowed to. I had been forced by circumstance to be a physician; to deal intellectually with my grandfather's ailments. He was just another patient. But this patient was my grandfather. A man I had loved dearly.

Conclusion

It was twenty-odd years ago that I first began medical school. And looking back over these past two decades I realize that I have become increasingly cynical about the practice of medicine. And that saddens me. I had started off with typically idealistic notions about what being a physician was all about. And like all idealism it was inevitable that reality would have to intrude and replace it. But I didn't think it would happen so quickly, and so completely.

Like a cop too many years on the beat I sometimes feel like I've seen too much. Too many healthy patients complaining and whining. And too many patients dying. Too many people smoking and drinking. And then being stunned when they fall ill. Too many incapable colleagues. And too many other colleagues protecting them. Too much time acting like a physician. And not enough time simply being one. Too many games. Too many games.

It's not just me of course — sharing these experiences, that is. In fact, it is astounding how uniform things truly are. Whether I am talking to a colleague from Toronto or Los Angeles, Moscow or Paris, Hong Kong or Sydney, their experiences are mine. Their cynicism is mine. Their ups and downs, highs and lows are mine.

And their concerns for their patients are mine too. Like everybody else on this planet, physicians assuredly vary in the level of skill that we bring to the job, but I find it quite striking how with surprisingly rare exception, we genuinely care and care deeply at that, for the patients we serve.

Yes, perhaps it is just a game. And maybe I don't play the game any worse or any better than anyone else. But maybe, just maybe, enough good happens to enough people that this is a game worth playing after all.

So to hell with cynicism.

"Mrs. Smith, I'm Dr. Blumer. Let me show you into the examining room...."

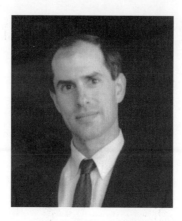

Ian Blumer, M.D. grew up in Montreal, attended medical school at Queen's University in Kingston, did his post-graduate training in Toronto and London, Ontario, and subsequently set up practice in internal medicine in Ajax. He has a subspecialty interest in diabetes and thyroid disease. Dr. Blumer and his wife (a rheumatologist) have three children.